AAK - 8102

Treating
Child Abuse
and Family Violence
in Hospitals

Treating Child Abuse and Family Violence in Hospitals

A Program for Training and Services

by
Kathleen M. White
Jane Snyder
Richard Bourne
Eli Newberger

FOREWORD BY
Saleem A. Shah

Lexington Books
D.C. Heath and Company / Lexington, Massachusetts / Toronto

Library of Congress Cataloging-in-Publication Data

Treating child abuse and family violence in hospitals.

"Based largely on work supported by grants from the Antisocial and
Violent Behavior Branch, National Institute of Mental Health
(TO1 MH 15517), and from the National Center on Child Abuse and
Neglect (90-CA-915A), Department of Health and Human Services. The
work was prepared under Research Training Grant T32 MH18265
from the National Institute of Mental Health"—T.p. verso.
Bibliography: p.
Includes index.
1. Child abuse—Prevention. 2. Family violence—Prevention.
3. Abused childen—Hospital care.
I. White, Kathleen M., 1940–   . II. National Institute of Mental
Health (U.S.). Antisocial and Violent Behavior Branch.
III. National Center on Child Abuse and Neglect.
IV. National Institute of Mental Health (U.S.)
[DNLM: 1. Child Abuse—prevention & control. 2. Family.
3. Hospitals, Special. 4. Violence. WA 320 T7837]
RC569.5.C55C74   1989   362.7′044   88-27034
ISBN 0-669-20822-1 (alk. paper)

Published simultaneously in Canada
Printed in the United States of America
International Standard Book Number: 0-669-20822-1
Library of Congress Catalog Card Number: 88-27034

The paper used in this publication meets the minimum requirements
of American National Standard for Information Sciences—Permanence
of Paper for Printed Library Materials, ANSI Z39.48-1984.

Year and number of printing:

89 90 91 92 8 7 6 5 4 3 2 1

Contents

Figures and Tables

Figures

Tables

Foreword

This work describes an innovative, exemplary program of training, research, and services for the treatment of family violence in a pediatric hospital, with a particular focus on child abuse and neglect. The report highlights critical conceptual and procedural issues, the limits of current clinical knowledge and related service needs, and various gaps between research and practice that must be addressed in the development and implementation of more effective hospital-based programs for the treatment of family violence. This monograph is based on the experience of an interdisciplinary training program, funded in 1979 by the National Institute of Mental Health's Antisocial and Violent Behavior Branch, in which postdoctoral clinicians and academic researchers were trained for interdisciplinary collaborative studies relevant to the understanding and treatment of family violence.

Among the conceptual and clinical innovations embodied in the program run by Dr. Eli Newberger and his colleagues is the view that child maltreatment is a family problem and that a whole host of childhood medical problems can most usefully be conceptualized as "pediatric social illnesses" with familial, child developmental, and environmental antecedents. This view helps to shift clinical and treatment attention away from an exclusive reliance of acts and perpetrators, or on symptoms and sanctions, to a more productive concern with familial and environmental causes and various points of intervention. Moreover, this program has long recognized the critical importance of training—beyond the bounds of particular specialties and disciplines—as a means of bridging the gap between empirical research and clinical practice, and providing better-informed and more effective services to victims of intrafamilial violence.

The setting for the training program, Children's Hospital in Boston, reflects the reality that medical services are frequently the first (and sometimes only) point of entry into the human services system for victims of family violence. Centering the program at this regional pediatric facility, which has been a major teaching resource for the Harvard Medical School, also reflects the belief that pediatric hospitals have important roles and responsibilities in the family violence area, including the training of clinical and research professionals and the development of specialized services. In the training program, clinicians have learned to design and conduct—by themselves and in collaboration with trained scientists—high-quality research on questions of importance to their own clinical work and interests; similarly, behavioral and social scientists have been oriented to the importance and necessity of conducting research in those clinical settings where their findings can more readily be translated into practice.

We are pleased to make this research available to a wide audience of program directors, clinical practitioners, and clinical researchers and trainers in children's and general hospital settings; to clinical and research faculty in graduate schools of nursing, psychiatry, psychology, and social work in connection with training in the area of family violence; to mental health, social service, and protective care personnel at state and local levels; and to academic researchers in the behavioral and social sciences. We hope that this book will be useful in the development of improved services for the prevention and treatment of family violence.

—Saleem A. Shah, Ph.D.
Chief, Antisocial and Violent
Behavior Branch
National Institute of Mental Health

Preface

D ealing with family violence is no easy task. Within medical
settings, the urgent need for acute medical care can make
it particularly difficult to deal with the social and environmental
contexts within which family violence is embedded. Moreover,
medical personnel often have little training in handling ambigu-
ously defined problems for which there are no simple procedures
or drugs.

Several years of experience at Children's Hospital Medical
Center in Boston have made it clear that a training program in
family violence can do a good deal to counteract the frustration
and pain that come with the attempt to address problems of family
violence in a hospital setting. This experience is shared in this book,
which is intended to inform, educate, and encourage hospitals,
related health delivery systems, and mental health and social service agencies to develop and/or strengthen their own programs and
activities in the area of family violence. The book should also be
of interest to state and local social service, child protection, and
related agencies, as well as to graduate training programs in various
mental health disciplines.

A paradox arises in the treatment of family violence in medical
settings. For the most part, hospital personnel are oriented to the
treatment of symptoms; unfortunately, if the underlying causes of
family violence are not addressed, the symptoms recur. Hospital
staff typically do not have the wherewithal to deal with such issues
as unemployment, or the subcultural or societal values that facilitate
acceptance and promotion of violence as a legitimate way of solving
human conflicts. Moreover, the family violence field has a way of

wearing down even the most optimistic and energetic professionals. An effective training program can provide a continuing source of intellectual stimulation and valuable experience that can offset some of the sadness and futility that seem inevitable when trying to help victims overcome the sometimes insuperable obstacles of the medical, social work, and legal bureaucracies.

With the development of a training program at Children's Hospital, work with cases of family violence became easier. Members of the hospital staff were increasingly congenial to the Trauma X (child abuse) treatment team. Colleagues also become more responsive to issues raised in consultations about particular cases and in teaching conferences about family violence. By providing tools for improved understanding and service interventions in regard to family violence, the program led to more active and sensitive involvement on the part of individual hospital personnel and diverse specialty units.

Our experience also showed that even a rather small initial core of dedicated medical practitioners can establish extremely productive cooperative relationships with social service personnel and behavioral scientists. Armed with persistence and intellectual excitement, such practitioners can open the doors of the teaching conferences, which are normally restricted to members of the hospital's medical staff. Teaching conferences and case discussions can be used to address the larger contextual issues of family violence. With such exposure, professionals can gain a clearer sense of what can be done when, for example, they are facing problems related to the status of women in marital conflicts or addressing alcoholism and other substance abuses. With consideration of these broader issues, medical practice pertaining to family violence can be improved.

In addition, in-service education can stimulate all participants with new knowledge, varied clinical and research approaches, and the complementary perspectives of people from different disciplines. A rich process of exchange can be set up. Hospital staff can learn from behavioral scientists and social service personnel. These professionals in turn can broaden and deepen their understanding of human behavior and of clinical work within a medical setting.

We acknowledge with deep appreciation the contributions of our colleagues whose support enables us to continue our work in this field: Helen Berkley, William Bithoney, Lisette Blondet, Roy Bowles, Jessica Daniel, Barbara Danzell, Howard Dubowitz, Debby Fenn, Amy Garber, Richard Gelles, Robert Hampton, Drew Hopping, Daniel Kessler, Sylvia Krakow, Joanne Michalek, Carolyn Newberger, Tim Schuettge, Stephen Shirk, Betty Singer, and Pamela Whitney. We also extend our thanks to the members of the staff of the Antisocial and Violent Behavior Branch at the National Institute of Mental Health, and of the National Center on Child Abuse and Neglect, whose guidance was always welcome and was frequently invaluable; we especially acknowledge the contributions of Aeolian Jackson, Thomas Lalley, Saleem A. Shah, and Ecford Voit.

Treating
Child Abuse
and Family Violence
in Hospitals

1
Why Family Violence Is
an Important Area

In the course of time Cain brought to the Lord an offering of the fruit
of the ground, and Abel brought of the firstlings of his flock and of
their fat portions. And the Lord had regard for Abel and his offering,
but for Cain and his offering he had no regard. So Cain was very angry,
and his countenance fell. . . .

Cain said to Abel his brother, "Let us go out to the field." And
when they were in the field, Cain rose up against his brother Abel, and
killed him.

Cain and Abel, those well-known biblical figures, were
brothers; the violence between them represents just one of
the forms that family violence can take. Brother can fight with
brother, sister with sister, spouse with spouse, parent with child,
child with parent—and conflicts between any pair of family
members are likely to be embedded in more widespread patterns
of violence and neglect.

The type of family violence usually seen within a pediatric
hospital or clinic is what is commonly called child abuse.
Moreover, much of the literature in the field of family violence
focuses on the maltreatment of children. However, considerable
evidence shows that focusing on child abuse to the neglect of the
more general problems of family violence leads not only to over-
simplified conceptions of the issue but also to short-sighted clinical
solutions.

Sometimes when children are brought to medical settings with
injuries that clearly were inflicted, blame is placed on a sibling.
Trying to determine whether the sibling really inflicted the injury
may distract clinicians and other involved professionals from the

larger task of determining what in the family circumstances explains why violence is occurring and just how generalized the violence is. Consider three cases seen in just one day at Children's Hospital.

Nancy, a one-and-a-half-year-old girl, was admitted through the emergency room because of burns to the head and fingers. Examination revealed healing burns on one hand and old scratches and bruises scattered over her body. Her "social" admission was linked to the various symptoms of abuse. After a 51 + A (child abuse report) was filed by the hospital, it was learned that her seven-year-old brother had been in foster care until about six months earlier, that the family was an open Department of Social Services case, and that the brother's stay in foster care stemmed from an earlier care-and-protection decision based on evidence that he had been burned and neglected. The brother was considered to be a seriously disturbed firesetter, and apparently he had been alone with Nancy when she received the head and finger burns. Clearly, an effort to determine whether the brother had inflicted Nancy's latest burns does little to address the multiple problems facing these children, and indeed the entire family.

Admitted on the same day was Nora, an eight-year-old girl allegedly raped by her sixteen-year-old brother. Conversations with the mother revealed that she had been concerned about this boy's sexual interests for about two years. Indeed, she and the boy's older sister had visited a psychiatrist to express their concerns—and had been told that his behavior was just a normal part of adolescence.

While the rape of an eight-year-old child might seem to some family violence experts like clear evidence of parental neglect or of putting a child at risk, the parents in this case seemed appropriately concerned and anxious for help. With the support of a social worker, the mother called all the neighborhood families for whom the boy baby-sat and said that he would be unable to work for them anymore because he was "having problems." A psychiatrist specializing in sexual abuse took the boy into therapy, and arrangements were made for psychiatric help for the raped daughter. Social services input, as needed, was also made available to the parents.

Malcolm, a nine-year-old boy, was admitted with amputation of a fingertip while away overnight at camp. There was no question of an inflicted injury in Malcolm's case; indeed, superficially the injury seemed very much to be an accident. However, Malcolm's family was known at Children's Hospital because a younger sister had been admitted several months earlier with a diagnosis of failure to thrive.

An investigation into the family circumstances revealed that Malcolm had been placed in the summer camp by a social service agency that wanted to give him a good summer experience and to get him away from parents who were seen as neglectful and as failing to supervise him. While at Children's Hospital, Malcolm was seen by a psychiatrist who characterized him as needy and hostile and as having difficulty with relationships. Malcolm's "accident" appeared to be symptomatic of his failure to protect himself in a family of five children where most of the parenting was done by Malcolm's twin sister. Calling Malcolm's injury an "accident" while labeling some other child's injury "abuse," though technically correct, would mean ignoring the whole host of common factors in the two situations, and perhaps in both cases failing to identify the kinds of family interventions that might help safeguard the futures of these children and their siblings.

These brief vignettes illustrate several points: (1) things are not always what they seem; (2) relying on a determination of parent culpability as a way of neatly classifying injuries as "inflicted" or "accidental" may not be the most useful appproach to the circumstances surrounding the injury; and (3) a focus on the injury per se rather than on the circumstances in which the injury is embedded may result in failure to address those underlying problems—so that nothing is done to alleviate the probability of repeated medical problems. Newberger et al. (1977) pointed out that a number of childhood medical problems ("pediatric social illnesses") have a "social" (generally family) component in their etiology. Included within this category—along with accidents and failure to thrive—are child abuse and neglect. However, differentiating among the various pediatric social illness diagnoses may not be as important as recognizing that familial/environmental issues may need to be addressed in all cases. Careful evaluation often uncovers a broader constellation of violence and/or neglect, or of circumstances putting other family members, as well as the pediatric patient, at risk. Important findings concerning pediatric social illness can be found in "Child Abuse and Pediatric Social Illness: An Epidemiological Analysis and Ecological Reformulation," appendix A of this book.

Violence as a Family Problem

Conceptualizing domestic violence as a family problem rather than focusing more narrowly on child maltreatment has many implications for both researchers and practitioners. Behavioral scientists seeking to understand the etiology of child abuse need a systemic perspective: consideration of the two parents and their relationship, of all family members in relation to each other, and of the family in relation to neighborhood and broader social institutions. Similarly, if one is concerned with the effects of the family environment on the child, including the possibility that observing violence will affect the child's behavior, then a systemic conception of the family is indeed essential. (The possibility that children can be victimized by observing rather than directly experiencing violence must be considered.)

Forms of Child Abuse

Because the abused or neglected child is often the "identified victim" who brings a multitude of family problems to light, the rest of this chapter focuses on the types of cases most likely to be seen in pediatric practice. As covered by the mandatory reporting laws, "child abuse" refers to physical and emotional abuse and neglect, medical and educational neglect, and most recently, sexual abuse and exploitation. In the course of evaluating and treating a range of problems—including accidents, ingestions, failure to thrive, and any number of medical conditions—medical and social service personnel may discover evidence of one or several of these forms of abuse. Moreover, other members of the family, including parents and grandparents, may be victims as well as victimizers in a cycle of violence and neglect. In each of the following examples of the major types of child abuse cases seen at Children's Hospital, it should be clear that focusing only on the symptoms of the child patient means neglecting a whole host of related problems.

Physical Abuse

Greg was a three-year-old admitted with a spiral fracture (that is, a fracture giving evidence of twisting) of the right leg. He also had a healing fracture of the right arm (that is, a fracture incurred earlier), and multiple bruises on the face, head, arms, chest, back, buttocks, and ears. Examination also revealed an old fracture of the left seventh rib.

Greg was the older of two children living with a divorced mother and her boyfriend. At the time of admission, the mother reported that Greg had fallen out of the car while it was moving and that she had fallen on top of him (while the boyfriend was driving the car). A friend of the mother's who called the hospital and asked to speak to a social worker reported that the boyfriend was violent, abused the children, and had been indicted for assault on a man whom he assumed had made a pass at the children's mother. When questioned by a social worker, the mother admitted that the boyfriend had abused both children severely but refused to alter her account of Greg's injuries.

Neither mother nor boyfriend went to see the child, who appeared very withdrawn, after his admission. Faced with strong evidence of physical abuse, the hospital filed a 51+A and a care-and-protection petition, and both children were placed in foster care.

Greg's case was somewhat atypical in that the evidence of abuse was clear-cut and witnesses to incidents of abuse were available and willing to testify. Despite these circumstances, Greg had been admitted by referral from a small community hospital where physicians were convinced of abuse but did not want the responsibility of filing a child abuse report. Indeed, the process of entering the legal/judicial system with cases of abuse is not typically relished by the individuals and agencies involved.

Child Neglect

Neglect of children can be broadly defined as failure to provide for or meet their emotional and developmental needs, including the need for adequate nutrition, clothing, shelter and safety, intellectual stimulation and education, and health and dental care. The problem is more omission of care than commission of injury. When such a broad definition is adopted, all parents may appear at times to fall short of meeting a child's many needs. However, the question of neglect arises when lack of parental care appears to be jeopardizing physical or emotional well-being or interfering with development.

Child neglect seems to be more pervasive than the physical abuse of children. When harm to a child is severe enough to require hospitalization or medical attention, it is one and a half times more likely to be due to neglect than to physical abuse (American Humane Association 1981). Data from the National Reporting Study indicated that 63 percent of all reported cases of child maltreatment involve "deprivation of necessities," while emotional maltreatment accounts for 14 percent of all reported cases of child abuse.

Neglect is often associated with abuse, and medical practitioners may see expressions of both problems in the same children. Martin (1980) noted that children who have been physically injured by their caretakers are also more likely to have received inadequate medical care, including lack of immunizations; moreover, their illnesses, such as ear infections, often go untreated. He also reported a higher incidence of undernourishment and anemia among physically abused children. Similarly, Newberger et al. (1977) reported that victims of physical abuse are more likely to be underweight for their age and are less healthy than children with other diagnoses.

Melissa was a one-year-old admitted with low weight gain and failure to thrive. She had gained only three pounds since birth. Both parents alleged that Melissa had not gained weight because she was difficult to feed; however, they also admitted to giving her frequent laxatives although they had been told by clinic staff not to do so. In the hospital Melissa appeared ravenous. The child's medical record revealed that the mother had a history of resisting and breaking medical appointments for the child. Also of concern was Melissa's three-year-old brother, who had also been seen for failure to thrive and who showed no normal language development.

When the hospital's Trauma X (child abuse) team evaluated Melissa, they concluded that the only apparent basis for the failure to thrive was parental neglect and failure to feed her; there was simply no evidence of any organic condition. On the basis of this diagnosis, a care-and-protection petition was filed, and the court awarded full temporary custody to the state Department of Social Services.

While this action was seen as fully appropriate by the Trauma X team, several nurses believed that the parents behaved in a warm and caring manner with their child, and that the legal action was inappropriate. Such disagreements are not uncommon among staff members who are unequally trained in issues of child maltreatment. Indeed, one of the difficulties associated with addressing issues of family violence and neglect is such disagreement among observers.

Sexual Abuse

The sexual abuse of children by adults has been labeled the "last frontier" in child maltreatment. It is the form of maltreatment most recently discovered by the pediatric community and society at large—although, as was the case with physical abuse and neglect, historians have noted its occurrence for centuries (DeMause 1974). Sociologist David Finkelhor (1979b) noted that the "discovery" of this social problem was facilitated by the women's movement, which brought the problem of rape and sexual abuse of women to public consciousness, leading in turn to awareness of the sexual victimization of children.

In the area of sexual abuse, as in other areas of family violence, it is important to have clear definitions. Although some people (for example, members of the Man-Boy Love Association) argue that sexual relations between adults and children can be "good" for, and enjoyed by, children, any sexual interaction with a child that is undertaken for the sexual gratification of the adult should be considered exploitative and abusive. A judgment of sexual abuse is also appropriate when (*a*) children are exposed to or involved in sexual activities inappropriate for their developmental level; (*b*) children are exposed to or involved in sexual activities inappropriate for their roles in the family; and (*c*) children are unable to give informed consent because of age or power differences in the relationship.

Estimates of the incidence of sexual abuse vary. Gagnon's reanalysis of Kinsey's data on 1,200 adult women indicated that 28 percent had had at least one sexual experience with an adult prior to the age of thirteen (Gagnon 1965). (Gagnon's definition of sexual experience includes exhibitionism as well as physical contact, which is consistent with the criteria just listed.) Applying this rate to the population of girls under thirteen leads to an estimated incidence of 500,000 cases of sexual abuse per year. According to data from the American Humane Association, in 9,000 cases of sex crimes against children, 75 percent of the perpetrators were adults who were familiar to the child. In a recent study of almost 800 college students, 19 percent of the women and 8.6 percent of the men reported sexually victimizing experiences as children (Finkelhor 1979a). The most common sexual experience was genital fondling. For women, half of the perpetrators were family members; for men, family members constituted 17 percent of the perpetrators.

Reported victims of sexual abuse are primarily girls, who constitute 80 percent of the cases reported nationally (American Humane Association 1981). Surveys of adult women indicate that between 19 and 34 percent were sexually victimized during childhood (Gagnon 1965, Finkelhor 1979a). Finkelhor's data suggest that boys are victimized with greater frequency than had previously been thought. Based on several surveys of adult males, Finkelhor estimates that 2.5–5.0 percent of boys under the age of thirteen are sexually victimized each year. This estimate extrapolates to an annual national incidence of 46,000–92,000 abused boys. The number of cases of sexual abuse that actually are reported each year is considerably lower than projections such as Finkelhor's, which are based on retrospective self-report data. In 1979, for example, 7,600 cases were reported (American Humane Association)—which is probably considerably fewer than the number of incidents that took place.

Sexual abuse may be underreported to a greater extent than any other form of child maltreatment for a number of reasons. First, the frequent absence of physical sequelae to the victim means that cases do not come to the attention of health professionals to the same extent as cases of physical abuse or neglect. Second, children are reluctant to report sexual experiences, particularly when the offender is a parent or other familiar adult. In Finkelhor's study (1979a), 63 percent of the female victims and 73 percent of the males had not told anyone about their experiences. Third, professionals themselves deny the problems. Rosenfeld (1979) has sensitively discussed the strong emotions engendered by sexual abuse cases in health and mental health professionals.

Katie, a three-and-a-half-year-old girl was admitted with vaginal bleeding after her father allegedly removed a squirt gun from her vagina. While damage to the vaginal area was extensive, the emergency room physician believed that the injuries were compatible with the father's story; nevertheless, a 51+A was filed by a social worker in the emergency room. The child's mother requested that the social worker evaluate the eight-year-old brother. Plans were also made for the sexual abuse team to evaluate all family members. Both parents vigorously denied any involvement by the father in the child's injuries, and despite strong suspicions on the part of the sexual abuse team the evidence of abuse was insufficient to justify removal of the child from the home.

Jenny was a four-year-old admitted through the emergency room because of serious vaginal damage. Her distraught young mother reported that she had "given marching orders" to the man with whom she had been living. Before moving out, he had gotten her out of their apartment on some pretext, then raped Jenny (not his daughter). The man had since disappeared, and the mother did not know where he had gone. Although no one presumed the mother's complicity in the rape, some concern was expressed by members of the Trauma X and sexual abuse teams as to whether this mother could adequately protect her child.

Conclusions

Clearly, many children in our society are at risk of maltreatment through physical abuse, neglect, and/or sexual abuse. Often, but not always, the effects of such maltreatment bring these children to the attention of medical and social service personnel. Sometimes the symptoms of the maltreatment can readily be identified for what they are. More often, perhaps, the symptoms are ambiguous, and professionals may disagree as to whether maltreatment has taken place. Even when a child is clearly at risk in a particular family environment, the appropriate action is not always obvious. Evidence that is sufficient to convince hospital personnel that maltreatment has taken place is not necessarily sufficient for the judicial system.

Child maltreatment, like other forms of family violence, has been recognized as a social as well as a medical problem. As such, it has received attention from social and behavioral scientists desiring to understand the problem, as well as from clinicians faced with making decisions about how to deal with its effects. In the chapters that follow, we consider both researchers' findings about family violence and the barriers to using research knowledge in hospital settings.

2
Conceptual and Procedural Challenges Facing Family Violence Service Programs

Michelle, a one-year-old girl, was brought by her parents to the emergency room because of an ear infection and a suspected seizure. Derek, ten-year-old son of divorced parents, was referred to the hospital's Family Development Clinic by the attorney for his mother, the noncustodial parent, who was seeking to regain custody from an allegedly abusive father. Are Michelle and Derek the victims of child maltreatment? Who should make this judgment? When is the evidence of abuse sufficient to justify the filing of a child abuse report? Who decides that the evidence is sufficient? What kind of evidence is appropriate? Is it enough to have a lack of fit between the nature of the child's injuries or overall condition and the parent's explanation of the problem? Is it useful or relevant to inquire about the family's general living situation, current concerns, and so forth? And again, who decides?

In this chapter, we present the argument that in each of these cases family problems were being expressed as symptoms in the children who were brought to the hospital for care. In each case, judgments about whether maltreatment had taken place were influenced by conceptions of the nature of child maltreatment and its etiology. Conceptions of child abuse that are incomplete or in some ways incorrect can lead to incorrect diagnoses—assuming child abuse has taken place when it has not, or missing cases of child abuse when they appear. Indeed, viewing child abuse as a simple matter of gruesome injuries inflicted on a helpless child by a "sick" parent, while popular, neglects much of what we have learned about family violence. Before presenting the cases of Michelle and Derek in more detail, we discuss major views on child abuse and family violence which influence the handling of such cases.

Conceptions of the Problem

Efforts to identify the characteristics of "child batterers" began with the identification of "battered" children by Kempe and his colleagues (Kempe et al. 1962). In this approach, children are seen as victims and parents as victimizers. From this perspective, it is appropriate to try to define the characteristics of "child abusers" (for example, Fischoff et al. 1971) and to treat the child abuse by excising the malignant agent—that is, by putting the parents in jail or in other ways making it impossible for them to inflict further injury on the child.

Since the publication of the Kempe paper, a number of efforts have been made to develop screening inventories (for instance, Milner and Ayoub 1980, Paulson et al. 1975) for identifying potential or actual child abusers. However, although some circumstances in people's lives may increase the likelihood of child maltreatment, there is strong evidence that only a few abusing parents show severe neurotic or psychotic characteristics; indeed, child abuse may be associated with several different parental personality types (Smith et al. 1975).

The assumption that child abuse is the product of parental psychopathology is quite consistent with what Sarason and Doris (1968) and other social scientists have called the *medical model*. From this perspective, the etiology of a problem like child abuse is mental illness, and the focus of intervention efforts is on treating the sick parent—for example, through psychotherapy. In the medical model, we would expect to see medical practitioners addressing the medical problems of the child, and social workers and psychiatrists dealing with the parent's presumed psychopathology—unless, of course, the judicial system intervenes. Although this approach may seem to work in some medical institutions, it is not responsive to the complexity of the problem of family violence and thus leaves many of the contributing problems unaddressed.

Family violence generally, as well as child abuse more specifically, is often conceptualized by social scientists as the product of poverty and/or stress—and here the concerns are quite different from those of the medical model. From the perspective of this *stress model*, all individuals caught up in the cycle of family violence are victims, even if only the child bears the scars of inflicted injury or neglect. Social scientists subscribing to this approach see little sense in trying to identify the personality characteristics of child abusers; they believe, instead, that almost any individual can become violent toward other family members if placed under enough stress. The solution to family violence, then, is to address the problems of poverty, unemployment, chronic illness, and so forth, which give rise to the violence. Although substantial empirical evidence may support a link between stress and violence, this link may seem irrelevant to medical practitioners who see the correction of social ills as legitimately outside their area of concern and expertise. Familiarity with the stress model may nevertheless influence the interpretations brought to a particular case of child maltreatment by clinicians—particularly social workers, who see such problems as falling within their domain.

Substantial evidence, some of which is reviewed in chapter 3, shows that neither the parental psychopathology nor the stress/poverty model is sufficient to account for the problem of family violence. Characteristics of the parent, characteristics of the child, characteristics of the situation (for example, level and type of stress) all appear to contribute to the likelihood that various forms of family violence may take place. Indeed, a *systemic model* of family violence, in which the potential role of a range of interrelated factors can be considered, appears to be a much more valid and useful approach to the problem. Such a model was developed by Newberger and Bittner (Bittner and Newberger 1981) and can be found in chapter 3, along with a review of the research supporting different elements within the model. For further discussion of the limitations of unitary models of child abuse and the advantages of a systemic approach to family violence, see Newberger and Newberger (1982).

Case Vignettes

Let's return to the cases of Michelle and Derek and see how conceptions of family violence and issues of training and turf affect the response of hospital personnel to children at risk.

Michelle

One-year-old Michelle was brought to the emergency room by her parents. According to the history taken from the parents, who were young and described by the social worker as "appropriately concerned," Michelle had been healthy until two weeks before the visit when she developed an upper respiratory infection, with congestion and nasal stuffiness. One day prior to her visit to the emergency room, the child was noted by her parents to be feverish and sweating. She vomited once. As was the usual practice, she had been taken by the mother into the parents' bed and nursed. At about 4:30 A.M., she woke crying and rolled off her parents bed onto a carpeted floor, hitting her head. She cried immediately, and her father put her back into her crib, at which time she appeared to be fine. Approximately half an hour later, Michelle suddenly became tense all over her body and appeared not to be breathing. This episode lasted about thirty seconds, after which she was again responsive. The parents thought Michelle's eyes had deviated toward the left during the episode. The child was taken to the emergency room in a local hospital where an ear infection was diagnosed. She was sent home with a decongestant and an antibiotic, and the mother gave her one dose. She remained feverish, and at 11:00 A.M. the father heard a noise from the child's room. Michelle was found to be twitching all over for about thirty seconds, following which she was dazed for about five minutes and then returned to normal. At this point she was taken to the emergency room at Children's Hospital. While there, she had another seizure, which consisted of the twitching of her left arm and the deviation of her head to the left. In the emergency room the child was seen by a house officer and a pediatric neurologist. A social worker was called to speak with the parents, who were obviously upset.

The following information was obtained. Michelle had had an unremarkable birth history, and her development and growth appeared normal. She had fallen from her parents' bed on at least three or four occasions and had sustained a total of seven or eight falls since she was four months of age. At four months she had fallen out of her crib when her parents, not suspecting she could roll, had left the side rail down. The most recent fall had occurred when she fell down six stairs after she had opened a gate. Though she had hit her head on a number of these occasions, no medical attention had been sought because Michelle always looked well following the incident. The mother did, however, note these events carefully in her baby book.

On examination, Michelle looked healthy and was obviously well cared for. She had no bruises and no outward sign of trauma. The parents were supportive of each other. Michelle responded well to her parents and was easily comforted by them. The parents reported that the child was left-handed and had been so for months. A careful examination revealed that the child had a preferential reach with her left hand and that her right hand and foot were definitely smaller than the left.

A seizure in a child with a high fever is not uncommon. However, typically these seizures are generalized; they do not show laterality (the predominance of motor activity to one side or the other). This child's seizure was unusual because it showed evidence of a focus that was left-sided and not generalized. A discharge of activity in the right side of the brain was causing head, eye, and hand motor movements to the left. In addition, the lesion causing the activity appeared to be old, because of the early onset of "handedness" on the left; moreover, the difference in size between the left and right extremities indicated damage to the nervous system that was not of recent onset.

During their interview with the social worker, the parents were openly tearful and frightened. They appeared unconcerned about the number of falls the baby had sustained and openly shared information about the early stresses in their lives and the father's recent feelings of anxiety and depression. The father volunteered information that he had previously had violent rages toward his wife, but that he had brought these under control when he started therapy—when Michelle was about four months of age (the time of her first fall).

How are we to understand a case like this? Is Michelle simply an unlucky, or perhaps "hyperactive," child who has managed to fall prey to a number of chance "accidents" and a fever-inducing ear infection? Is the principal responsibility of hospital personnel to diagnose and treat the fever, or should they determine whether some form of parental failure to protect and nurture their child may have contributed to the child's history of repeated falls—a history that on the surface appeared unrelated to presenting symptoms of fever and seizure? What should be done if, as became evident in Michelle's case, the medical and social service staff cannot agree as to whether an injury or medical condition reflects troubled family dynamics or just a simple, ordinary, everyday type of accident?

To some extent, the referral of Michelle's case to the Trauma X consulting team was accidental. The social worker on duty when Michelle was brought to the emergency room was a member of the Trauma X team who was covering for another social worker. This Trauma X team worker became concerned over the social history of the family and the repeat accidents to which the child had been prone. The medical staff, particularly the young house officer on duty that night, interpreted the case as being exactly as presented—an ear infection that had led to a fever and minor seizures. This house officer saw no need for a Trauma X consult. However, the social worker did see a need, and the process was set in motion.

What was the physician's perception of Michelle and her family? "Kids will be kids, all kids have accidents," he said. In Michelle's parents he saw two college graduates who owned a nice home in the suburbs and two cars, parents who kept careful records of their child's development, took her into their bed at night when she cried, and persistently sought medical help for her apparent seizures. How could abuse be suspected in such a nice middle-class family? In light of the literature on biases associated with the labeling process, it is not surprising that the physician refused to consider a diagnosis of maltreatment in this case.

What, on the other hand, did the social worker see when she talked with the family? She saw a father who admitted that he had beaten his wife until recently—indeed, right up until the time the baby's falls had begun—and who reported that he had been in therapy six years because he had trouble controlling his "rage." The social worker also saw a mother who did not want her in-laws to know that she and her husband were at the hospital with the baby because she was afraid her mother-in-law "will have the baby taken away." Moreover, while the mother was pleased to share her diary of Michelle's infancy, it was noteworthy to the social worker that medical advice or treatment had never been sought in relation to the repeat accidents reported therein.

Which perception was correct—the physician's or the social worker's? What is the proper way to proceed when one professional is concerned about possible threats to a child's health and safety and another professional is not—especially when there is a major differential in power and authority? In this case the social worker sought the Trauma X consult. The physician, miffed that the social worker took action that he deemed inappropriate, banned that social worker from further contact with the family so that she could "upset them" no more!

Michelle's case illustrates well a number of the difficulties encountered within medical settings by professionals responsible for diagnosing and responding to child abuse. Physicians tend to view injuries and illnesses as medical problems in need of medical treatments. Social workers sometimes see injuries and illnesses as psychological disturbances, family problems, or social realities in need of therapeutic intervention. Physicians have greater power and authority. Social workers generally are more subordinate, and they typically have less power and authority than members of the medical profession—especially in a hospital setting. Moreover, although roles are changing, physicians generally are men and social workers generally are women. Although gender, power, and prestige should be irrelevant to the goal of protecting children, in reality they can have a determinative effect. Who wins out when a young man with an M.D. after his name, freshly out of his internship though he may be, regards an experienced social worker as overly emotional, judgmental, and meddlesome? Whatever the merits of any particular case, it is unlikely to be the child who wins when titles rather than experience carry the day. Hospital legal staff are reluctant to pursue legal action on behalf of a child when their own professionals disagree about the merits of the case. Moreover, even when a case goes to court, the credentials of physicians may carry greater weight than the informed judgments of social workers—and again, the child may be the loser under these circumstances.

What was particularly unfortunate in Michelle's case was that social science knowledge on family violence supported the social worker's interpretation. Nevertheless, this knowledge became irrelevant in the political arena of actual decision making. Specifically, there was evidence of other forms of family violence (the father against the mother), a vulnerable parent who had a troubled relationship with his own mother and had been in therapy for years to help in controlling his rage, and considerable ongoing social stress, freely reported by both parents. All of these characteristics have been identified as contributing to the complex etiology of the multidimensional problem commonly known as child abuse. Further discussion of differences of opinion among professional groups concerning child abuse can be found in appendix B, "Consensus and Difference among Hospital Professionals in Evaluating Child Maltreatment."

Derek

The medical record for ten-year-old Derek, the child custody case, contained some important information about treatment administered to him at other hospitals on several occasions. For example, he had been x-rayed and treated on one occasion for fractured ribs. Another time he was treated for head injuries. In all instances, his injuries were treated and he was released to his custodial parent, that is, his father—not an atypical outcome when a child is brought to a medical setting by a parent for treatment of injuries. Little had been done about the fact that the fractured ribs evidently had been caused by kicks to the chest inflicted by Derek's father; nor had action been taken when head injuries occurred because Derek's father threw him against a wall.

When Derek's mother found out about her ex-husband's abuse of her son, she obtained a court order for temporary custody and an evaluation of Derek. In the ensuing Family Development Clinic evaluation, a chilling story of family violence emerged, a story that might never have been discovered in clinical settings focused only on healing injuries.

The oldest of nine children, Derek's mother married at age seventeen to escape an unhappy home in which her own father frequently abused her mother. Soon pregnant, she became the victim of her husband's regular physical beatings. Derek was born prematurely, was "always sick," and himself became subject to his father's violent assaults. When he was two, his mother left him in the care of her own mother. Distraught from her husband's abuse and his threats to shoot or stab her, Derek's mother admitted herself to a psychiatric hospital. Derek's father sought and won both a divorce and custody of his son from a judge who refused to talk to a boy who was unhappy and afraid about being placed with his father.

Derek's father continued beating him and a second wife, whom he married right after his divorce. The second wife also fled from the beatings, leaving her stepson behind. Ultimately, Derek's mother learned of the ongoing physical violence and sought custody of her son. On the basis of a thorough evaluation that confirmed the father's physical and emotional abuse of the child, the Family Development Clinic team recommended that the mother be given custody of her son and that Derek receive extensive psychological and educational services.

This story illustrates well the finding of social scientists (for example, Straus, Gelles, and Steinmetz, 1980) that child abuse frequently occurs in families where violence characterizes the spousal relationship. Derek's story is an emphatic reminder of the importance not only of looking beyond physical symptoms to their causes but also of avoiding a narrow conceptualization of child abuse. Often family violence envelops not just children but also adults, whose victimization may extend through many areas of their lives. Moreover, as a premature child with health problems, Derek can be seen as a good example of the vulnerable child described by researchers as susceptible to abuse from an early age. Finally, whatever his personal history or mental health status may have been, Derek's father, as a career military man, may have been particularly subjected to sociocultural pressures favoring strict discipline to enforce obedience.

As tragic as the case of Derek and his mother is, it has a relatively happy ending. Family Development Clinic personnel, as well as representatives of the judicial system, concurred that Derek should be placed in the custody of his mother and that the family should receive helping services. Such unanimity is by no means commonplace among the professionals who deal with family violence. Moreover, interventions on behalf of children and their families do not always serve those who are the most in need—for example, the mother whose inability to protect her child is linked to her own victimization. A discussion of factors influencing decisions concerning the disposition of child abuse cases can be found in appendix D, "Returning Children Home: Clinical Decision Making in Cases of Child Abuse and Neglect."

Responding to Family Violence Cases

As illustrated in these vignettes, cases of family violence create special problems in the medical settings where they are seen. Public recognition of child abuse as a medical-legal issue and mandatory reporting laws thrust new responsibilities on physicians and other clinical personnel who continue, generally, to be ill-prepared to handle them.

If institutions are to deal adequately with child abuse and other forms of family violence, a number of general goals deserve attention. One major goal should be to develop an interdisciplinary team. Members of the different professions typically have different perspectives, conceptions, terminology, and professional tools, and also different status in service delivery and other settings. In light of the anger and frustration that can often be engendered when possible child maltreatment is being assessed, these differences can lead to and exacerbate problems in communication and in interpersonal relationships. Any institution undertaking an interdisciplinary team approach to family violence services must be prepared to cope with these problems. In later chapters we present a number of practical suggestions derived from our own experience for dealing with case management.

A second major goal should be the classic one of integrating research and practice—that is, of finding ways of making extant behavioral and social science research available and usable to practitioners. Our message, reiterated several times in this book, is that the institutions should provide opportunities for researchers and practitioners to work together and to communicate their particular knowledge, skills, and viewpoints. Seminars, journal groups, colloquia, and case conferences can all be useful, especially if considerable care and flexibility are devoted to the process involved in developing and conducting these opportunities for interchange.

Establishing vehicles for communication between researchers and practitioners can be an important antidote to the affliction that often keeps these groups of professionals on two different wavelengths. A number of reasons account for the current gaps between social science and clinical knowledge, and opportunities to close these gaps are likely to benefit everybody. Consequently, it is useful for developers of training programs to understand the reasons for the gaps and to address these reasons in planning.

1. *Lack of communication among social scientists and clinicians.* Professionals tend to publish and to read within their own discipline. "Keeping up with the literature" can be an awesome task even within one's own discipline. Professional training programs tend to be unidisciplinary and to draw heavily from a unidisciplinary literature. This narrow exposure is especially the case within the field of medicine. Medical schools and residencies continue to emphasize biomedical course work and training. They typically exclude course work on psychology, the family, and social problems from the required curricula—even in regard to issues such as family violence, which have direct consequences for medical practice.

2. *A difference in the construction of knowledge and criteria for significance.* Even when communication does occur between clinicians and researchers, each group—at an interdisciplinary conference, for example—is likely to feel that the knowledge communicated by the other is irrelevant or invalid. This paradigm clash between social scientists and clinicians was well described by Gelles (1982). The researcher is often concerned with finding the smallest number of variables that explain differences between selected

groups—for example, families in which violence occurs as compared with families in which violence appears to be absent. To the researcher, knowledge consists of accrued research findings that must meet standards of scientific validity such as adequate sampling size and techniques, use of control groups, and sufficient demonstration that the results are statistically significant—that is, they could not have occurred by chance.

The goal of the clinician, on the other hand, is to understand the individual case, to identify a particular problem, and to determine which of the clinical factors contributing to the problem are amenable to intervention. Knowledge consists of accrued experience with families or individuals, which might be categorized into types of families and problems, and knowledge of what does and does not work.

Factors of *clinical* significance might be different from factors of *research* significance. For example, though researchers might argue that parental alcoholism occurs in only a small percentage of family violence cases and is not a significant contributor to family violence *in general*, the clinician may be faced with individual families in which parental alcoholism appears to be a highly significant factor.

3. *Mutual skepticism.* Because of differences in training, in construction of knowledge, and in work roles, clinicians and researchers often feel mutual skepticism concerning each other's contributions to knowledge and to issues raised within the area of family violence. Researchers may assume that clinicians are not critical enough of the generalizations they make on the basis of their experience with cases and may dismiss the case study approach as nonscientific. Clinicians may assume that researchers are not aware of the real world and may dismiss research findings as too simplistic or irrelevant because they fail to capture the many variables operating in the lives of families or those that are amenable to change.

This lack of communication and mutual mistrust is a serious impediment to effective collaboration. Researchers may continue to design studies that fail to address issues of greatest significance for clinicians. Clinicians, meanwhile, may continue to generalize from their experience without the benefit of checking this very selected or biased experience against research findings with non-clinical samples and control groups.

Conclusions

In many hospitals, clinical practice with cases of family violence continues to be guided by conceptions focusing narrowly on child abuse. Emphasis remains largely on parental psychopathology as the cause of maltreatment and on the parent as villain rather than another victim. Moreover, a symptom-oriented approach continues to guide medical practice, with insufficient attention given to the psychological and social dimensions of the case. The latter is particularly true for physicians, who, as a group, are in a position of authority for decision making and case management in hospital practice. Hence, the biomedical approach may predominate amidst conflict with nurses and social workers more attuned to psychosocial issues.

The implications of these shortcomings for families and children are serious. Cases of violent, neglectful, or sexual maltreatment may be missed completely, or additional family victims may fail to be identified, and children and families may fail to receive the protection and services they need. Biases in recognition and reporting of cases according to race and socioeconomic status are also likely to occur. The myth that family violence is a problem only of poor people or of those very different from the professionals themselves continues to influence practice. Also, conflict among disciplines in case management, when cases are identified, may be the norm. An inadequate understanding of what causes family violence and a lack of agreement on how to manage such cases may result in inappropriate or insensitive intervention with families.

Now more than ever the need for training in this area is critical. Pressures on families, such as unemployment and financial stress, are increasing as helping resources are diminishing. Hospital emergency rooms increasingly become the gateways into the service system for families in trouble, as other doors have closed. Timely and sensitive intervention into the family processes behind the presenting symptoms may help prevent future hospital admissions and even save lives. It is essential that hospital professionals be knowledgeable about and prepared to deal with a number of components that can be adopted in other settings. Of particular importance is allowing some time away from a demanding schedule to review and reflect on one's work with families and the questions generated by colleagues and others offering different but useful perspectives. Although one's own assumptions and biases may be challenged in an unsettling way, new information and perspectives can also lead to intellectual and professional growth. Before describing the major components of our own training program and making recommendations for training in other settings, we review, in chapter 3, research evidence concerning family violence which has implications for practitioners and which could be made available to practitioners through an interdisciplinary training program.

3
What Is Known about
Family Violence

The concept of the sanctity of the family has a long history. Traditionally, families have been regarded as a refuge for their members. Within families, individuals are presumed to care for and take care of each other. We now know that however rosy a picture may be painted of families in our folklore or in our popular media, family members can actually be a source of harm to each other.

This chapter provides a brief overview of what is known about family violence. We focus particularly on those products of family violence most likely to be seen in pediatric settings—that is, children who have been physically or sexually abused and/or neglected. After summarizing what is known about the incidence of family violence, we review the research literature on the etiology of various forms of child maltreatment. The effects of violence and sexual abuse on children, the preferential labeling of certain groups of children as abused or neglected, and the effectiveness of different kinds of intervention in cases of family violence are also considered.

Incidence of Family Violence

The true incidence of the various forms of family violence is difficult to determine. Statistics on the incidence of child abuse, for example, rely on figures from child protection agencies, which provide only the number of cases reported. Although the nationwide incidence of reported child abuse cases is known to have increased by 71 percent between 1976 and 1979 to a total of 711,142 cases (American Humane Association 1981), experts agree that this increase reflects both greater public awareness of this social problem and increased agency accountability rather than a rise in true incidence of child maltreatment.

A landmark study of the incidence of family violence was published in the book *Behind Closed Doors* by Straus, Gelles, and Steinmetz (1980). These sociologists surveyed a representative national sample of two-parent families with children between the ages of three and seventeen concerning the incidence of violence among family members in their household. Administered in the context of an interview was the Conflict Tactics Scale, which presents a sequence of methods of conflict resolution, progressing from benign means to increasingly violent acts, such as hitting, kicking, biting, or beating up, and ending with threats of or actual assault with a knife or gun. The results of the survey by Straus, Gelles, and Steinmetz (1980) are worth summarizing here.

Violence toward Children

The prevalence of severe violence directed toward three- to seventeen-year-old children was 3.8 percent in the survey year. One in every 1,000 children was threatened or assaulted with a knife or a gun. A projection of this ratio to the 46 million children aged three to seventeen who lived with both parents during the survey year suggests that 1.5–2 million children per year are threatened or assaulted with lethal weapons; 46,000 of those children are actually subjected to use of a weapon. In addition, 8 out of 100 parents reported using one of these forms of violence against a child one or more times in the child's life. Children experiencing lesser forms of violence—kicks, bites, and punches—suffered such events an average of 8.6 times during the survey year. Beatings occurred an average of once every two months.

Violence was not confined to young children. When analyzed by age group, 82 percent of the three- to nine-year-olds, 66 percent of the ten- to fourteen-year olds, and 34 percent of the fifteen- to seventeen-year-olds, had been victims of some form of violence during the year. Although the figures are high enough to be very disconcerting, they may actually be an underestimate of violence directed toward children by their parents. First, the data are self-reported, and many respondents may have denied or played down the use of violence in their homes. Second, omitted from the survey were two groups considered to be at risk for violence: children in single-parent households and children under three years of age. (These two groups of children have now been included in an NIMH-funded replication and expansion of the 1976 survey, currently being conducted by Dr. Murray Straus and his colleagues at the University of New Hampshire. This "Resurvey of Physical Violence in American Families" was scheduled to be completed in 1988.)

Interspousal Violence

Straus, Gelles, and Steinmetz also reported that one out of every six respondents (16 percent) admitted some kind of physical violence at the hands of the spouse during the survey year. Over the course of marriage, the chance appeared to be greater than one in four (28 percent) that a couple would engage in an act of spousal violence. Projected to the 47 million marriages in the United States, the data indicate that about 1.8 million women suffer severe physical violence each year. These data further suggest that a similar number of husbands are victims of violent acts by their wives. Also, women who experienced severe violence were 150 percent more likely to inflict severe violence on their children than women who did not.

Straus and Gelles (1986) have noted, however, that the meaning and consequences of wife-to-husband violence are easily misunderstood. The greater average size and strength of men and their greater aggressiveness mean that the same act (for example, a punch) is likely to be very different in the amount of pain or injury inflicted. Even more important, a great deal of violence by women against their husbands is retaliatory or in self-defense, since the risk of assault for a typical American woman is greatest in her own home. Nonetheless, "violence by women against their husbands is not something to be dismissed because of the even greater violence by their husbands" (Straus and Gelles 1986).

Other Forms of Family Violence

In the same study, the most frequent form of family violence was between siblings. Almost 5 percent of the children in the sample had made threats with or used a knife or gun against a sibling in their lifetime. Severe sibling violence was much more frequent in families in which parents were often violent toward their children or toward each other; specifically, sibling violence occurred in 100 percent of such households, as compared with only 20 percent of households in which parents did not use violence toward their children or toward each other.

Children who were victims of parental violence were more likely to use violence against the parents. Among those children who had been hit the most by their parents, 50 percent used violence in return. On the other hand, less than one in four hundred of the children who were not hit by either mother or father were violent toward a parent.

Strauss, Gelles, and Steinmetz (1980) found violence to be widespread among families. The study documented the occurrence of different forms of violence within the same families. Families in which interspousal violence occurred were more likely to direct violence toward children, and children who witnessed or were targets of violence were likely to be violent with siblings and parents.

The Causes of Family Violence

The etiology of family violence is complex. Violence is best understood as a symptom associated with the interaction of a number of factors in any given family. One must further take into account the particular vulnerabilities in a child, parent, or family that heighten their susceptibility to particular stresses that may in turn result in violence. Bittner and Newberger (1981) proposed a multidimensional etiological model of family violence, which is diagrammed in figure 3–1. This model summarizes predisposing factors in family violence, which can result from interactions among sociocultural factors and stresses operating at the levels of society, family, parent, and child.

No systematic study has been made of the events that precipitate abusive acts. Some instances are acute and self-limited; other cases are of long duration. Nonetheless, when maltreatment is evident in a child who has been brought to a medical setting for treatment, it is helpful to consider circumstances in the family's life immediately prior to the visit. Clinical experience provides examples of a number of situations that can trigger abuse: a baby who, on a particular evening, would not stop crying; an alcoholic father who was fired from his job; a mother who, after being beaten by her husband, could not contact her own mother; the serving of an eviction notice. Any one of these stresses could trigger violence.

As summarized in figure 3–1, a number of variables can interact in ways that lead to child maltreatment. Examples of each major category of variable are provided in the section that follows. Though the focus in figure 3–1 and the material that follows is on child maltreatment, the model is relevant to other forms of family violence as well. In all cases, violence is embedded in a family system that in turn is embedded in broader socioeconomic systems, and in all cases the violence is likely to stem from the interaction of multiple causes.

Child Factors: Vulnerabilities and Stresses

The realization that children as well as their parents shape the course of family interaction is a fairly recent insight (Harper 1975, Patterson et al. 1975). This perspective has led to the identification of children's characteristics that interfere with normal family functioning. In reviewing the literature on special characteristics of the abused child, Friedrich and Boriskin (1976) noted that behaviors that make children especially difficult to care for and

Social-Cultural Factors

Values and norms concerning violence and force; acceptability of corporal punishment
Inegalitarian, hierarchical social structure; exploitative interpersonal relationships
Values concerning competition vs. cooperation
Inequitable, alienating economic system; acceptance of permanent poor class
Devaluation of children and other dependents
Institutional manifestations of the above: law, health care, education, welfare, sports, entertainment, etc.

FAMILY STRESSES

Child-produced Stresses

Physically different
  (e.g., handicapped)
Mentally different
  (e.g., retarded)
Temperamentally different
  (e.g., difficult)
Behaviorally different
  (e.g., hyperactive)
Foster child

Social-Situational Stesses

Structural factors: poverty, unemployment, mobility, isolation, poor housing
Parental relationship: discord-assault, dominant-submissive patterns
Parent-child relationship: attachment problems, perinatal stress, punitive childrearing style, scapegoating, role-reversal, excess or unwanted childen

Parent-produced Stresses

Low self-esteem
Abused as a child
Depression
Substance abuse
Character disorder or psychiatric illness
Ignorance of childrearing: unrealistic expectations

Triggering Situation

Argument/family conflict
Acute environmental problem

Discipline
Substance abuse

Maltreatment

Inability to provide care
Psychological maltreatment

Injury
Poisoning

Adapted from Bittner and Newberger 1981. Copyright 1981 by *Pediatrics in Review.*

Figure 3–1. *Model for Understanding Child Abuse*

parental perceptions of the child as different or difficult have been associated with abuse.

Included among these special characteristics of abused children are physical handicaps, congenital physical disabilities, mental retardation, schizophrenia, neurological damage, language deficits, and hyperactivity. In addition, low birth weight and prematurity have been linked with abuse—perhaps because of early infant-mother separation or associated special characteristics, such as irritability. Excessive crying or fussiness is another characteristic of abused children. The causal relationship between abuse and developmental disabilities may be bidirectional: developmentally disabled children appear to be more vulnerable to abuse by caretakers, and abuse and neglect possibly result in developmental disabilities.

Parental Vulnerabilities

Parental psychopathology was assumed in the first clinical reports to be the single reason for child maltreatment. Indeed, if present, it may adversely affect a parent's behavior toward a child. However, less than 10 percent of abusive parents appear to be psychologically disturbed (Steele 1978). Two factors seem to be critical in determining how vulnerable a parent is to adopting abusive behavior toward a child: (1) the parent's ability to understand and empathize with the child, and (2) the parent's own history, including exposure to violence or deprivation in his or her own family of origin.

Research and clinical findings indicate that parents who use violence against their children were frequently subjected to violence as children (Newberger et al. 1977, Parke and Collmer 1975, Straus, Gelles, and Steinmetz 1980). However, "not all parents who have experienced violence as children use violence against their children" (Straus, Gelles, and Steinmetz 1980). Thus, caution must be exercised in drawing deterministic conclusions from this association.

It also has been argued that parents who were physically abused as children were frequently deprived emotionally as well. Consequently, as adults they may suffer low self-esteem, depression, and feelings of powerlessness. To compensate, they may achieve goals through coercive tactics applied to those even weaker and less powerful than themselves—that is, to their own children.

Family Stresses

A number of researchers have described an impaired attachment relationship between parent and abused child. A healthy attachment requires reciprocal responsiveness to signals from each other. Factors impairing the reciprocity include perceptual handicaps, developmental disabilities, illness, or irritability on the part of either parent or child. Premature infants appear to be at greater risk for attachment difficulties (Klaus and Kennel 1976) and for later abuse than do full-term infants.

Other family factors implicated in child abuse include the absence of one parent through job demands, separation, illness, divorce, or single parenthood, and the social isolation of a family through lack of friends or relations nearby, distance from transportation, lack of a phone, or noninvolvement with the community (Newberger et al. 1977). Straus and his colleagues (1980) found that high numbers of stressful life events (eight or more) were strongly related to incidents of severe violence against children.

A major stressful condition for many families in which children are abused is poverty. Though some investigators of child and spouse abuse have claimed that socioeconomic factors were not related to acts of domestic violence, the very articles containing these claims offer empirical evidence that abuse is more prevalent among those of low socioeconomic status (Gelles 1981). Indeed, a number of studies of family violence support the hypothesis that such violence is more prevalent in low-income families (Parke and Collmer 1975, Gil 1970). Many other social stresses found to be associated with child abuse correlate with lower socioeconomic status, such as unemployment, poor housing, family size, and lack of access to child care (Newberger et al. 1977). However, this conclusion does not mean that domestic violence is confined to lower-class households (Straus, Gelles, and Steinmetz 1980, Gelles 1981).

Sociocultural Factors

Consensus is increasing on the association between the acceptance of violence as a normative means of socializing children and child abuse. The use of corporal punishment is widespread, and it could be argued that physical punishment of children expresses societal values in a familial context. Controversy reigns over the legal and moral legitimacy of violence toward children as well as other forms of family violence. The support of corporal punishment by such institutions as the United States Supreme Court appears to sanction violent practices in the American home even though some of these practices culminate in serious harm.

The depiction and promotion of violence in the movies and on television may also affect how adults and children approach conflict. Whether media violence is associated with childhood aggressive behaviors remains a subject for lively debate, but consensus is developing that a milieu of violence fosters actions of violence.

Poverty, not parental failure, is cited by Gil (1975) as the principal "abuse" of children, and its continuation as an example of "socially structured and sanctioned child abuse." Many poor children, reported as victims of child abuse and neglect, are placed in foster homes because serious economic and familial problems deprive parents of the resources that enable them to care adequately for their offspring. Too often those foster homes and institutions are also inadequate or even harmful.

Research on Pediatric Social Illness

An innovative approach to etiological research on family violence can be found in our work at Children's Hospital Medical Center in Boston (Newberger et al. 1977, Newberger, Hampton, and White 1986). Our clinical and research team has been interested in a variety of symptoms in children that appear to result from family psychosocial circumstances rather than from disease or mishap. These symptoms are associated with the diagnoses of household accidents, ingestion of toxic substances, nonorganic failure to thrive, and child abuse. It appears useful to consider those diagnostic categories as forms of "pediatric social illness" and to investigate the etiological similarities and differences among the four groups.

In our landmark study, a sample of children between birth and the age of four years was selected from each of the four pediatric social illness diagnostic categories and then matched with control subjects on the basis of age, race, and socioeconomic status. Data on parent, child, family, and social circumstances were gathered through a lengthy maternal interview. Considerable overlap in etiological factors was found, as well as some differences among the four groups. Families of child abuse cases differed from families in the other groups in the sheer number of stresses operating on them, and in the lower poverty level at which they were subsisting. A later cluster analysis (Newberger and Marx 1982) of pediatric social illness data produced three distinct groups: families enjoying "ecological advantage," families suffering from "ecological adversity," and families overwhelmed with "ecological crisis." Cases representing each diagnostic category, as well as control cases, were found in all three clusters. These data support the notion that family violence is one of several possible symptoms of family distress, and that all of the pediatric social illnesses are linked to family and environmental stresses. Later research on pediatric social illness can be found in appendix A.

Research on Sexual Victimization of Children

Child sexual abuse, which is just beginning to receive systematic study, has been defined as "the involvement of children in sexual activities that they do not fully comprehend, to which they are unable to give informed consent, or that violate the social taboos of family roles" (NCCAN 1981).

Because less than 50 percent of sexually victimized children have any physical symptoms, these cases must be identified through the children's behavioral and psychological indicators of distress or developmentally inappropriate sexual behavior. Despite the difficulties in identification, hospital emergency rooms are seeing increasing numbers of child and adolescent victims of sexual abuse.

Characteristics of Perpetrators

Individuals who sexually abuse children tend to be male. This finding occurs in both clinical and survey reports, with both male and female victims, and in both intrafamilial and nonfamilial abuse. In Finkelhor's study (1979a), 84 percent of the perpetrators were male; in the National Reporting Study, males were perpetrators in 86 percent of the cases of sexual abuse with male victims and 94 percent of the cases with female victims.

Data on convicted offenders distinguish between two types of male offenders involved in sex crimes against children: fixated and regressed (Groth and Birnbaum 1978). The fixated offender would appropriately be labeled a pedophiliac, for whom children are the primary and exclusive sexual object. For the regressed offender, the usual sexual choice is an adult female, but stress or a crisis in family relationships may lead to regression and the choice of a child or adolescent sexual partner. A third type of offender would be the indiscriminately promiscuous adult who chooses children and adults of either sex as sexual objects.

Adults who sexually abuse children are seldom psychotic and may appear perfectly normal to the observer (Summit and Kryso 1978). These offenders also tend to be familiar to the child as family members, friends of the family, neighbors, or baby-sitters.

Incest

The incestuous family has received considerable attention in the recent clinical literature, most of which has focused on father-daughter incest. As described by a number of clinicians (Summit and Kryso 1978, Weinburg 1955, Cormier, Kennedy, and Snagowicz 1962), the "endogamous incestuous family" appears on the surface to be quite normal but suffers from serious role distortion. In the relationship between the spouses sexual involvement becomes absent, and the father-daughter relationship becomes sexual. The involved daughter (usually an adolescent) is described as taking the role of the mother in many ways, because of the mother's withdrawal through illness, depression, or emotional unavailability. The father who engages his daughter in incest has often victimized the mother through violence, coercing her into a passive role. Lustig et al. (1966) described an implicit condoning of the incestuous relationship by the mother and the painful fears of separation and abandonment characterizing all members of the family. The incestuous relationship, it has been suggested, holds the family together. In some cases, however, the pattern is less organized and very promiscuous, with greater role confusion and more blurring of boundaries than in the endogamous family (Weinburg 1955).

Less commonly reported to child protection agencies are sexual relationships among siblings or stepsiblings. Survey data indicate that this may be the most common type of incest but the least harmful (Finkelhor 1979a, Nakashima and Zakus 1977). Incestuous sexual experiences are more likely to be repeated over a long period of time than are sexual experiences with nonfamily members (Greenberg 1979).

Issues of Definition and Labeling

As noted in chapter 1, current reporting statutes define child abuse broadly to include physical and emotional injury and neglect, educational and medical neglect, and sexual abuse. The responsibility of applying these labels to specific situations and behaviors is left to individual practitioners, protective service agencies, and the courts. Clearly, in applying a label such as child abuse and judging the deviance of a parental practice, ambiguous definitions can lead to selective labeling of minority or disadvantaged groups. Turbett and O'Toole (1980) demonstrated that when the same case vignette was presented with ethnicity or income status altered, a difference in diagnosis occurred, with minority and lower-income children most likely to be labeled as victims of child abuse.

A recent secondary analysis (Hampton 1983) of data from a national study of the incidence of child maltreatment also revealed dramatic racial and class bias in actual reporting practices in hospitals. Race and class, but not medical severity, significantly discriminated those cases reported to protective service agencies by a sample of seventy hospitals in the ten states participating in the study.

Difficulties in diagnosing child abuse may also stem from differences among professionals in evaluating the seriousness of the impact of certain parental practices on the children. Giovannoni and Becerra (1979) studied the amount of consensus and difference among professionals and found that they distinguished among kinds of maltreatment and generally agreed as to the relative rank ordering of particular parental behaviors in the seriousness of their consequences for the child. However, significant differences in absolute ratings for degree of seriousness existed among professional groups. Giovannoni and Becerra concluded from their data that greater precision in legal and clinical definitions of child abuse would greatly aid practice in this area.

As long as ambiguity in definitions of child abuse and neglect persists, the problem of biased labeling and professional differences in judgment will lead to preferential diagnoses of abuse and neglect based on criteria other than the characteristics of the caretaking situation itself. Through this process, some families may be subjected to intrusive protective measures when they are not called for, while children in other families may continue to be at grave risk with no intervention provided.

Effects of Maltreatment on the Child

The effects of physical violence and neglect on the child depend on the child's age and developmental level at the time of the event, the frequency and nature of the experience, and the total emotional milieu in the home. Few well-designed follow-up studies exist, and longitudinal data on the effects of physical abuse and neglect on children are extremely limited. From available clinical observations, however, it appears that physical violence and neglect affect a child at a number of levels, including physical, cognitive, and emotional development. Furthermore, Friedman and Morse (1976), in following up a sample of twenty-four abuse and neglect victims, found that in more than 70 percent of the cases, siblings had been injured as well. Research on each of the major areas of negative outcome is summarized briefly below.

Developmental Delay

Numerous studies of abused or neglected children provide evidence of delays in the areas of cognitive, language, and motor development. More severe developmental disabilities are also common (Martin 1980, Solomons 1979). Caffey (1972) warned that shaking infants can result in subdural hematomas that, if left untreated, can lead to mental retardation. A number of studies report that mental retardation in abused children appears to be a direct result of head trauma (Buchanan and Oliver 1979).

Emotional Impairment

Follow-up studies (for example, Kinard 1980) of victims of abuse and neglect suggest that the emotional tasks most impaired by aversive conditions in the home are the development of a positive self-concept, the management of aggression, and the development of social relations with others, including the ability to trust. Moreover, children who have been physically victimized or neglected by a caretaker are likely to feel that they are bad, unlovable, and unwanted. Physically abused children are frequently somber and unhappy, unable to enjoy activities, and rate themselves negatively on self-concept scales (Martin and Beezley 1977, Kinard 1980).

Aggressiveness

Physically abused children were reported to be more physically aggressive with peers than were comparison groups (Martin 1980, Martin and Beezley 1977, Green 1978, Reidy 1977). Neglected children were also rated as more aggressive than controls by their teachers. Green's data suggest that aggression is also likely to be turned against the self among abused and neglected victims. The possibility that abuse experienced as a child may be associated with later violent or delinquent behavior has been a long-standing concern. While Carr (1977) discovered evidence of considerable violence in the childhood histories of delinquent boys, the survey conducted by Straus, Gelles, and Steinmetz (1980) also showed clearly that not everybody who was abused as a child becomes an abusing parent.

Abused and neglected children often develop poor relations with peers and adults (Martin and Beezley 1977, Kinard 1980). In a study of fifty physically abused children, Kinard (1980) noted an active avoidance of peers and difficulty in giving and receiving affection in relation to parents and peers. Attachment behavior between abused and neglected children and their parents has also been found to be aberrant, including displays of indiscriminate attachment to adults and/or avoidance of the parent (Schneider-Rosen et al., in press).

Effects of Sexual Abuse on the Child

A number of factors determine the psychological sequelae of sexual abuse in the child, including (1) the nature of the sexual activity, its frequency of occurrence, and the use of force; (2) the age and developmental status of the child; (3) the relationship between the child and the perpetrator; and (4) the family's reaction.

Short-term effects of sexual abuse vary with the age of the child but include feelings of anxiety, mistrust, guilt, anger, fear, and depression. Behavioral symptoms may include regressive behaviors (enuresis, encopresis, crying, clinging), difficulties in school, withdrawal from peers, and acting out behavior that is sexual, aggressive, or self-destructive (Rosenfeld 1979, Simrel et al. 1979).

Summit and Kryso (1978) reported that victims of incest tend to suffer further sexual assaults from other family members following disclosure, and tend to blame themselves, suffering from depression and impaired sexual relationships in later life. Although some claim that sexual abuse is not necessarily harmful to children, knowledge of child development and the imperfect clinical evidence to date suggest that this argument lacks validity.

Information on the long-term effects of sexual abuse is extremely limited, and no systematic longitudinal data on childhood victims of sexual abuse exist. The only available information has been obtained from clinical reports, largely retrospective in nature, which show that children who have experienced single incidents of sexual abuse by a strange adult and are supported by their families seem to suffer fewer long-term effects, although short-term effects occur and must be dealt with. Children abused by family members for a long time, however, usually have less family support available following disclosure. Indeed, the child may be viewed as a traitor, responsible for "breaking up the family." If forced to testify in court, such a child must bear the burden of guilt for complicity in the sexual activity, disrupting the family, and possibly sending a family member to jail. Hence, in these cases it is difficult to separate the long-term effects of sexual abuse from the disturbed family dynamics and the aftermath of disclosure of the sexual activities.

Spouse Abuse

The literature on spouse abuse, like the literature on other aspects of family violence, is characterized by competing definitions and points of view. Most of the research focuses on wife abuse, which appears to be by far the more prevalent problem. Parker and Schumacher (1977) defined wife abuse or battering as a "symptom complex of violence in which a woman has, at any time, received deliberate, severe, and repeated (more than three times) demonstrable injury from her husband with the minimal injury of severe bruising." Though this definition implies that to qualify as abuse the husband's behavior must leave some evidence on the woman's body after the incident is over, other theorists (for example, Weitzman and Dreen 1982) consider any kind of physical violence, with or without bruising, as abusive. Similar definitions have been proposed that do not specify gender of victim and perpetrator.

The "discovery" of wife abuse as a social problem appears to have occurred in the 1970s with the rise of the women's movement (Pfouts and Renz 1981). Though previously viewed as a psychopathological, sadomasochistic marital relationship of concern only to the particular parties involved, wife abuse has more recently been defined by feminists as a problem "not of the individual but of a patriarchal society in which men held disproportionate power over valued resources and in which women were subservient to men both within the marriage and in all important facets of society" (Pfouts and Renz 1981).

Also, although wife abuse was initially considered to be a problem of the lower socioeconomic classes (Goode 1971), research now demonstrates that wife abuse crosses all socioeconomic strata (for example, Straus 1977–78). Powered by the feminist movement, recognition of the pervasiveness of wife abuse has led to stronger legal support for the rights of abused women and to programs designed to help the abused wife (Nichols 1976, McShane 1979, Costantino 1981).

The research literature on wife abuse contains at least two major perspectives: the personological and the sociological. Personological research is oriented toward describing the personality types of individuals who engage in violent relationships. For example, Ponzetti et al. (1982) suggested five characteristics of the male abuser:

1. Inexpressiveness

2. Alcohol and drug abuse

3. Emotional dependence

4. Difficulty with assertiveness

5. Personal experience with family violence—either as observer or victim

Moreover, for the personologist, abused wives share similar characteristics with their abusive husbands, including childhood histories of family violence, dependency conflicts, and a narrow range of coping responses (Weitzman and Dreen 1982). Abused wives have also been viewed as victims of "learned helplessness," having acquired early in childhood the belief that men and not their own behaviors control their lives (Walker 1977–78).

The personological approach to spouse abuse can lead to a focus on such characteristics of abused wives as a sense of incompetence and unlovableness, guilt and shame, and a pervasive sense of hopelessness (Hilberman and Munson 1977–78). The sociological approach, by contrast, starts with the premise that violence is a normal feature of contemporary society, not just a problem for a particular type of wife (for example, Goode 1971, Gelles 1974, Straus 1977–78). Goode (1971) noted that patriarchal social systems are based on an unequal distribution of power, and that in the family, as in other power systems, the threat of force underlies all interactions. Unequal power roles have become so internalized in family members that some wives report that they believe it is acceptable for a husband to beat up his wife every once in a while (Gelles 1976).

The recognition of wife abuse posed a recurrent question: Why do abused wives remain in abusive relationships? Gelles (1976) pointed to three factors that influence the abused wife's decision to seek help: (1) the less severe and the less frequent the violence, the longer a wife remains with her husband; (2) the more a wife was struck as a child by her parents, the more likely she is to remain with her abusive husband; and (3) the fewer resources and the less power the wife has, the more likely she is to stay with her husband.

Straus, Gelles, and Steinmetz (1980) provided strong documentation for their view that wife beating is part of the way of life for American families. They also noted, however, that violence between husband and wife is not a one-way street. Although husbands perform almost all types of violent acts more often than wives do, wives are more likely than husbands to kick or hit with objects. Straus and his colleagues suggested that differences between husbands and wives in violent behavior may be related more to the smaller size, lower weight, and lesser muscular development of most women than to any greater rejection of physical force on moral grounds. Neverthless, they concluded that wives are victimized by violence in the family to a much greater extent than are husbands and consequently should be the focus of remedial efforts.

What Interventions Work Best?

Little is known about the interventions that work best with families needing protective services. The interventions currently available include individual psychiatric treatment for violent family members, family treatment, parent education, and provision of day care, homemaking, and other concrete services. Efforts to prosecute parents who severely abuse (physically or sexually) their children have also increased recently.

A federally funded three-year evaluation of eleven service projects (the National Demonstration Program on Child Abuse and Neglect) by Berkeley Planning Associates, though methodologically flawed, provided some provocative data (Cohn 1979). "Severe reincidence" of abuse occurred in 30 percent of the families served while the families were in treatment. Reincidence was lowest when well-trained workers handled intake and treatment planning. In addition, serious reincidence was most likely to occur in those families in which the initial abusive incident was most serious, indicating that such families were in particular need of highly trained workers and intensive services. Another noteworthy finding was that workers thought that the potential for future mistreatment was reduced for only 42 percent of the clients served. When service programs were compared, the percentage of "successes" as rated by workers was highest for those clients receiving lay services such as Parents Anonymous, a lay counselor, or parent aide.

In her report on the National Demonstration Project Evaluation findings, Cohn also noted the relatively low rate at which children under the care of protective agencies received therapeutic treatment, despite the frequency of behavioral maladjustment. Kinard (1980), in a more systematic study of the effects of abuse on children's emotional status, also made a strong plea for systematic therapeutic attention for abused children. Finally, in professional decision making about intervention in families in which child maltreatment has occurred, the need for interdisciplinary collaboration was noted by many (for example, Newberger and McAnulty 1976, Bourne and Newberger 1980, Giovannoni and Becerra 1979).

Limitations to Research Evidence

Though knowledge in the area of child maltreatment and family violence has expanded considerably since the work done by Kempe and his colleagues (1962), the field is still in its infancy (Gelles 1980). Replicated studies are few, and theory remains rudimentary. We know more than we once did about incidence and some of the factors associated with family violence, but we still cannot explain why some families with these characteristics are violent or neglectful toward their children and some are not. Research on sexual abuse is in the early stages, and well-designed studies on the long-term effects of violence and sexual abuse of children are rare. Moreover, well-designed intervention studies are virtually nonexistent.

Current models of the etiology of family violence are complex and difficult to implement or test through research, which of necessity must limit the number of factors studied at any one time. The implications of these behavioral and social science etiological models for clinical practice are also complex. Identification of many levels of causation implies that intervention or prevention efforts at any one level, such as that of the individual parent, may not be sufficient.

Although available information about family violence has implications for clinical practice and policy, much is still unknown. Unfortunately, current findings fall far short of providing adequate answers to some of the questions of greatest interest to clinicians (for instance, those concerning the best intervention strategies and the effects of maltreatment on children).

Service Needs

Given the widespread incidence of family violence, health and mental health practitioners, as well as educators, will inevitably encounter children and families in whose lives family violence is a reality. How will professionals recognize these social problems and the need for intervention? What will they do when they encounter family violence and believe that intervention is necessary? How will they deal with the family, with their own difficult feelings, and with other professionals who become involved with the family?

Working in this area of clinical and professional practice is extremely difficult. Feelings run high, and action is often lacking. Moreover, failure to recognize the problem can have profound implications for the welfare of the children. Territoriality among professionals in these cases can be an added and serious complicating factor. Clearly, any training that promotes the sensitivity and the ability of the professional to recognize and deal effectively with these cases, to work well with other professionals, and to feel confident that the choice of intervention is based upon a secure knowledge base would be of great value. In the chapters that follow, we describe our own experiences at Children's Hospital, with the goal of helping professionals at other institutions develop effective ways of dealing with family violence.

4
The Children's Hospital Program on Family Violence

C oncern with the problem of child maltreatment began at the Children's Hospital in the mid-1960s, in response to the passage of a mandatory child abuse reporting law in Massachusetts. At first, Children's Hospital, like other medical facilities, was ill-equipped to deal effectively with the new responsibilities imposed by the law. Moreover, there was a critical shortage of personnel in the Department of Public Welfare, which was the state agency designed by law to receive reports of child abuse cases and to provide protective services. Thus, although individual physicians reported cases of inflicted injury to the Department of Public Welfare, the resources available to provide protective services were severely limited. The rate of reinjury in children whose cases had been reported appeared quite high to all observers, and the hospital personnel as well as Welfare Department staff agreed that a more systematic program of case finding, evaluation, intervention, and follow-up was essential.

In the 1969–70 hospital year, the financial and human costs of child abuse were measured through a study of length and expense of hospital stay and frequency of reinjury to children. So great was the cost and so high the reinjury rate that a review of existing knowledge and programs throughout the United States was undertaken. Cities such as Denver, Los Angeles, San Francisco, and Pittsburgh were visited to see the programs that had been developed in response to the passage of mandatory reporting laws in other states. In some of these settings, most of the responsibility for dealing with cases of child maltreatment rested in the hands of social service personnel, with physicians largely out of the process. Cities where physicians were more actively involved in the child maltreatment programs appeared to have a more effective approach.

The Trauma X Team

As a result of such observations, Children's Hospital developed a hospital-based child abuse consultation unit that included representatives from community-based social services organizations—for example, the Massachusetts Society for the Prevention of Cruelty to Children and the Department of Public Welfare. This interdisciplinary, interagency consultation unit, the Trauma X team, was formed in 1970.

The euphemism, Trauma X, defined as "a syndrome with or without inflicted injury in which a child's survival is threatened in his or her home," was adopted with the specific intention of focusing on risk to the child. We preferred this focus to a punitive concern with a family that was having difficulty providing adequate protection and/or nurturance for the child. Our adoption of the term *Trauma X* rather than, for example, *battered child* was just one expression of our general emphasis on violence and neglect as problems of family systems rather than as attributes of pathological parents. Outsiders might argue that the Trauma X team clearly deals with cases of abuse and neglect, but viewing these children as the products of family violence, which may also take other forms less often seen within the pediatric medical setting, fits better with our general philosophy.

To assess the impact of the new child maltreatment management system, costs were compared of treatment before and after formation of the Trauma X team. The data revealed that the average length of hospital stay decreased from twenty-nine to seventeen days after formation of the team; moreover, the injury rate declined from 10 percent to 1.7 percent. Setting up the team undoubtedly had other salutary effects as well, such as heightened institutional visibility for problems of family violence. Further information about reductions in "the literal and human cost of child abuse" following the introduction of the Trauma X management system can be found in Newberger et al. (1973).

Research and service programs associated with the child abuse consultation process were at first supported in part by a grant from the Office of Child Development in the Department of Health, Education, and Welfare (OCD-CB-141). The hospital later assumed the salaries of Trauma X team members originally supported on grant funds as well as other personnel yet to be described (such as family advocates, certain Family Development Clinic staff). Currently, between 125 and 150 cases of maltreatment are reported to the Department of Social Services each year. The Trauma X program now operates under the sponsorship of the hospital's administration, with a view to fostering strong collegial relationships among the participants. Cooperative relationships have developed among the hospital's Social Services Department (which numbers fifty workers), the members of the Trauma X team, the hospital's Office of Legal Counsel, and public and private family service agencies.

Ongoing research conducted by the child maltreatment program staff reveals that the Trauma X team continues to perform a vital function for the hospital and community. A record review of 280 Trauma X cases seen between 1978 and 1981 revealed that 201 (71.8 percent) of these cases were admitted through the hospital emergency room. Another 68 cases (24.3 percent) were transferred from other hospitals or outpatient clinics and either admitted or seen on an outpatient basis only. These Trauma X cases included 29 children (14 percent) with bruises, 37 children (18 percent) with burns, 25 (12 percent) with skull fractures, 21 (10 percent) with bone fractures, 25 (12 percent) with head injuries, and 26 (13 percent) with poisonings, as well as other problems. The severity of injuries ranged from fatal in 3 children (.01 percent) through life threatening in 30 children (15 percent), serious in 97 children (48 percent), moderate in 116 children (38 percent), and minimal in 31 (15 percent) children. Eighty percent of the children were under five years of age; 50 percent were under one-and-one-half years.

Child abuse reports were filed on 57.5 percent of the cases seen by the Trauma X team. Only 16.8 percent of the cases on which the team consulted were discharged to their homes without being provided with services from the Department of Social Services. Of the remaining children, 57.8 percent went home but were provided with services, 5.1 percent were placed in foster care with a relative, 15.2 percent were placed in foster care with a nonrelative, and 2.7 percent went into residential treatment. In more than 25 percent of the Trauma X cases, care and protection petitions were filed by either Children's Hospital or another agency involved with the family.

The Family Development Study

The clinical experiences of the Trauma X team at Children's Hospital led to the creation of a family violence research center, the Family Development Study. The focus of this research program has been on pediatric social illnesses—that is, on those childhood medical conditions that have familial, child developmental, and environmental antecedents. Child abuse and neglect, accidents, poisonings, and failure to thrive all meet these conditions. Together, they account for a major share of the mortality of preschool children, and each of them often has significant psychological and physical sequelae.

Much of the work of the Family Development Study has been motivated by the desire to help develop a national and universal classification system that would focus on both causal characteristics and direct treatment and intervention more appropriately and effectively than has previously been the case. For example, the roles of the child and the environment are typically overlooked in family violence cases when a disproportionate reliance is placed on harmful acts and perpetrators. Moreover, clinical approaches to accidents, poisonings, and failure to thrive are often limited by implicit conceptual models of chance occurrence, as implied by the names of these conditions. These diagnoses serve to direct clinical attention and treatment to the child's physical symptoms, while the familial and environmental antecedents and concomitants of the symptoms are ignored.

In order to develop a more adequate illness classification system for these social illnesses, members of the Family Development Study research team designed a controlled epidemiologic study in which 560 mothers were interviewed and medical data on their children were reviewed. Pediatric social illness cases and control group families were matched on age, ethnic status, and socioeconomic status. The data from several analyses support the central hypothesis that these social illnesses are related and that their common etiology includes important elements of stress in the family before, during, and after the birth of the child. (For more information, see Newberger et al. 1977, Bowles, Newberger, and White 1985.)

The Family Advocacy Program

A Family Advocacy Program was an important outgrowth of the work of the Family Development Study. When designing the interview to assess such stressors as limited access to essential services and general social isolation, the research team was faced with an ethical dillemma: could the pressing problems that were likely to be discovered then be ignored? Our group decided to accept this responsibility. Consequently, when interviewing for the Family Development Study began in December 1972, a family advocacy program was also instituted. By working to assure access to essential services such as housing, health care, child care, education, and legal aid, the family advocates endeavored to improve the environmental circumstances in which childrearing was embedded and to foster the optimal functioning of participating families.

The Family Advocacy Program appeared to be an extremely useful innovation. By working with parents around specific environmental and social problems, the advocates helped them develop a sense of personal efficacy and control. The parents began to see themselves not as passive victims but as active agents better able to control and deal with their own children. Through home visits, telephone calls, and office visits, the advocates developed personal and intensive contact with families and were thus able to help them in numerous direct and indirect ways, for example, persuading a landlord to restore heat or helping families obtain affordable legal aid. The Advocacy Program, like the Trauma X team, helped both to increase the visibility of child maltreatment cases and to orient attention to the more general problems of family violence.

In 1986 a new advocacy program began at the hospital. Called Advocacy for Women and Kids in Emergencies (AWAKE), it is a unique model of mother-child public health intervention in cases of family violence. (Our thanks go to Lisa Gary, director of the AWAKE program, for supplying us with this information.) As far as we know, it is the only program in the nation in a pediatric setting that provides dual advocacy for both battered women and their abused children.

Traditional pediatric practice in abuse cases has focused on child protection, failing to consider potential violence against the mother and, in fact, frequently blaming her for "failing to protect" the child. As a result, children have been removed from their homes and placed in foster care, but they can be victimized in these settings as well.

The basic premise of the AWAKE program is that professionals need to broaden their view of child abuse to include intervention on behalf of potentially battered women and to unite the services presently offered separately and conflictingly to women and their children. At Children's Hospital, an advocate works with a woman to prevent further and more serious abuse, to keep children out of unnecessary foster placement, and to refer mother and child to resources where they can receive help together. Services include court, police, housing, and welfare advocacy, support, and referrals.

The AWAKE project is based on the assumption, corroborated by several studies, that in 30–40 percent of child abuse cases there is also a battered woman. By mobilizing advocacy services on behalf of the mother, the staff assume they can help her keep her children. To date, fewer than five children have been placed in foster care. In an informal survey of twenty-four children served, twenty-one are with their mother (two were placed in foster care and then returned to their mother); two are with their mother and presumed abuser; two are with other relatives (one because of the mother's death); and one is with the abuser.

Since AWAKE began receiving referrals in October, 1986, it has provided advocacy and consultation to more than 150 women and 250 children. Services have ranged from direct advocacy to consultation with hospital staff and community groups. In addition, AWAKE has provided training to hospital staff, increasing their awareness of violence against women and providing them with guidelines for interviewing battered women and referral information.

AWAKE currently has two components: a hospital service and model development program and a public policy initiative. The hospital service and model development program, established through funding from a Victims of Crime Act grant (VOCA), combines professional child advocacy with self-help battered women's advocacy at Children's Hospital, Boston.

The public policy initiative, funded through the Boston Foundation, is supporting an examination of services, laws, and child protective policies affecting battered women and their abused children, studying what is provided, where the gaps are in service provision, and what the policies and guidelines are governing these services. This information is being used not only to create a more comprehensive program at Children's Hospital but also to develop more effective child care strategies within state agencies. To effect this change in policy and service, the hospital proposes to establish a pilot advocacy unit in an area office of the Massachusetts Department of Social Services (DSS). This advocacy project will replicate the model used successfully at the hospital.

The following case vignette illustrates the impact of AWAKE and highlights some of the problems we have tackled.

Mrs. Z and Mr. G had been involved in a relationship for over two years and had a fourteen-month-old son named Paul. Mr. G's violence escalated sharply and classically over time, culminating in a brutal, life-threatening beating of Paul, which necessitated restorative surgery and two and a half months of recuperation at Children's Hospital. During the first six weeks of Paul's hospital stay, although there was concern that his mother was being beaten by his father, no referral was made to AWAKE.

Mrs. Z was viewed by staff as uncooperative, because she would not say that Mr. G was the batterer, and at times she was observed holding hands with him in the waiting room. At other times, she asked staff to make him leave the hospital. Some nurses believed that she responded well to her son, whereas others expressed anger that she didn't visit him often enough. This ambivalence appeared to confuse, frustrate, and divide the staff. A month into hospitalization, Mr. G assaulted Mrs. Z on hospital grounds. Mrs. Z courageously described this attack to her DSS (child protective) worker and to a hospital social worker. Both told her to try to stay away from Mr. G.

Soon thereafter, the hospital social worker requested the assistance of AWAKE advocacy in this difficult and dangerous situation. With the AWAKE advocate, Mrs. Z mustered her strength and revealed again that Mr. G. had assaulted her. The advocate, well acquainted with these cases, responded to Mrs. Z in a supportive and understanding way, suggesting that they work together toward protecting Mrs. Z and her son. Mrs. Z reacted positively to this alliance and went to court with the advocate to secure an order of protection, and she arranged with hospital staff to bar Mr. G from visiting the hospital. Despite the strong conviction on the part of DSS and hospital social workers that Mrs. Z was unable to protect herself and her son, with the support of the AWAKE advocate Mrs. Z retained an attorney, fought for custody, and moved in with her relatives pending more permanent housing arrangements. With the advocate's help, Mrs. Z finally has felt safe enough to say that Mr. G did batter her and her son and has decided to be a witness in criminal proceedings against Mr. G for the violent abuse of Paul.

This vignette illustrates many of the issues in a dual case of woman battering and child abuse: initial primary focus on the child's medical and social condition; the mother's seeming ambivalence toward (or fear of) her partner, which confuses staff, causing them to blame her; the mother's need for intense, nonjudgmental support, which staff directly involved in the care of a severely injured child may not be able to provide; feelings of inadequacy and hopelessness in child protection and hospital social workers, causing them to look beyond the mother (to the foster care system) for the care of the child; constant interdisciplinary collaboration (with legal counsel and other staff) to protect both the child and mother and to find them housing, welfare and child care resources; and the need for strong advocacy for the mother, without which she may be immobilized and misjudged.

The Family Development Clinic

An outpatient clinic, the Family Development Clinic, was set up in 1972. This clinic specializes in the interdisciplinary assessment and treatment of children who present various physical and behavioral symptoms indicating that they are at risk of abuse or neglect. The clinic was designed to serve several functions: (1) to provide continuing aftercare services following hospitalization to pediatric social illness cases whose physical conditions had warranted inpatient treatment; (2) to divert children from hospital admission when, despite urgent family crises that might signal the potential usefulness of a "social admission," the children could be sustained safely in their homes; and (3) to organize the specialty resources at the hospital more effectively to deliver services to multiproblem families, and to consult with nonmedical professional personnel involved in their care.

The core staff for the Family Development Clinic consists of medical personnel (generally two pediatricians and a nurse practitioner), a social worker, and a psychologist. As part of their training, other personnel (for example, pediatric and psychiatry residents, visiting behavioral scientists) may rotate through service on the clinic team. The clinic staff regularly hold planning meetings every Wednesday afternoon and see patients Thursday afternoons. Other meeting times are arranged when patient schedules demand it.

Referrals to the clinic come from a variety of sources, including the Department of Social Services and the juvenile court. Generally, the clinic is asked to conduct a full social-psychological-medical evaluation to determine whether the child has been the victim of abuse or neglect, and to make recommendations concerning custody and services. All evaluations are conducted by an interdisciplinary team, composed typically of at least one medical professional and one social service professional, with the frequent inclusion of visiting professionals interested in problems of family violence. Often, additional information is sought from other institutions where the child—and perhaps the parent—has been seen. Further assessments may also be obtained from specialists such as neurologists and psychiatrists within the hospital.

An overview of Family Development Clinic intakes between July 1, 1981, and June 30, 1982, provides some useful information about the children seen by this outpatient service. In this one-year period, eighty-two children were evaluated. Sixty-two percent of the children were under five years of age, 24 percent were less than two years old. The basis for the referrals included suspected neglect, physical abuse, sexual abuse, and emotional abuse. Often, personnel from schools or courts had determined that evaluations were necessary not simply because of overt signs of physical abuse but because of such characteristics as excessive thinness and apparent malnutrition, self-abusiveness, severe behavior problems, developmental delay, or poor hygiene. As part of the evaluation and recommendation process, clinic staff spent time not only in the clinic but also in courts, schools, other medical settings, and the clients' homes. Though many of the cases were of a first-time nature, others had been coming to the clinic for evaluation and referral for years.

Development of a Clinical Training Program

The establishment of the Trauma X team and Family Development Clinic represented an important response to one manifestation of family violence as it appears in the pediatric medical setting. However, the core professionals involved in these two units became convinced that additional steps were necessary to improve the handling of child maltreatment cases at Children's Hospital and to contribute to general knowledge about family violence as well. The concern of these core professionals (a pediatrician, an attorney/sociologist, a social worker, and a nurse practitioner) stemmed from the high incidence of family violence cases at the hospital. The physical symptoms of child maltreatment and other forms of pediatric social illness could appear in any medical context. Having consultation units available was not sufficient if other hospital personnel did not recognize and respond to such symptoms in their patients. It was clear that broad professional education was essential so that practitioners in a variety of specialties would know how to interview families regarding questionable symptoms and how to interpret the information they obtained.

To meet the needs for training in family violence, the core group of family violence professionals at Children's Hospital obtained support from the National Institute of Mental Health (NIMH) for a clinical training program: the Model Hospital-based Training Program on Family Violence. A major element of this training program was in-service education, an effort that was already well under way when grant support was obtained.

Because in-service education is both an essential task and one that can be accomplished without external funding, we describe our own teaching program in detail here. Since the experience of the pediatric, psychological, and sociological fellows has implications for all efforts to improve family violence training through an interdisciplinary training approach, their experience and the implications of their experiences for training are also discussed.

In-service Training

The in-service education program was aimed primarily at pediatricians because that group appeared most focused on the treatment of physical symptoms and least responsive to the more general problems in which family violence is embedded. The content of training sessions was designed to be somewhat specific to the discipline addressed, but also to include a review of the psychosocial factors implicated in the etiology of family violence. Attention was given to the concept of child abuse as a subsidiary form of family violence, the problems of labeling among poor and ethnic minority families, the related problems of "missed" or undiagnosed maltreatment cases among middle- and upper-class families, and the need for prompt recognition of cases to facilitate careful decision making in case management.

When the training program was initiated, the project directors had already participated in in-service training at a number of different institutions. For the current project, each of the relevant clinical chiefs was contacted to arrange teaching on family violence. All training directors (and some chief residents) were informed of the objectives of the program. This undertaking involved a careful and diplomatic effort to engage the clinical services, whose emphasis has traditionally been biomedical, with little or no attention to psychosocial issues. Each department already had its own special teaching exercises and training techniques, and these had to be respected as cross-program cooperation was enlisted.

Another priority of the program was to obtain access to the conferences that had active participation by the senior staff and members of the visiting medical community—for example, grand rounds on the medical, orthopedic, and surgical services. It was hoped that persuading senior professionals of the value of multidisciplinary approaches to family violence would increase the likelihood of achieving the goals of the program. Many of these senior professionals, specialists in their own fields, were understandably reluctant to embrace programs that appeared to mean taking on broader responsibilities for ensuring the welfare of children and addressing psychosocial issues traditionally outside their areas of expertise. Thus, approaching these services was a delicate and difficult task, involving personal visits and gentle persuasion. The effort was more than worthwhile, for the chiefs of medical services typically had a tremendous influence on the junior staff, often serving as "ego ideals" whom the young physicians wished to emulate. In teaching hospitals where the emphasis is on training in technical skills, it is very important to convince senior staff of the value of serious attention to family issues. When senior physicians do not think it useful to talk to families, they find other things for their interns and residents to do, thus denying these trainees experience in dealing with families and communicating the view that talking to families about their problems is unimportant.

In the departments of social work, nursing, and psychiatry, there was generally greater acknowledgment of the significance of understanding family violence for clinical training. As part of their own training, professionals in these areas typically had been oriented to a concern with interpersonal issues and to an understanding of the importance of family relationships for the well-being of the individual. Consequently, the program staff encountered less difficulty engaging members of these departments in the training program. Indeed, the challenge was to strengthen the role of these professionals—particularly in the female-dominated professions of nursing and social work, which are often looked down upon by physicians.

In addition to enlisting the involvement of senior medical staff, people in this program made an effort to educate the pediatric trainees on issues of family violence. At Children's Hospital, as at many other training hospitals, junior medical personnel are loosely grouped into two categories: interns and residents. Interns are usually recent graduates of medical school. Residents generally have one to five years of postgraduate clinical experience; several in each training year have more extensive clinical or investigative backgrounds. About 40 percent subsequently elect careers in clinical practice; the other 60 percent go on to subspecialty training and academic work, which frequently involves both research and teaching.

In teaching hospitals, the junior staff have the actual contact with families. Thus, it is important for interns and residents to have the knowledge and practical skills to work effectively with families. They need to realize that certain symptoms may mean that further investigation is desirable. For example, if a child with a fractured leg is visited by a mother with a black eye, physicians should consider the possibility of family violence and not just confine themselves to fixing the fracture.

We assumed that by addressing pediatric fellows directly and relatively early in their training, we could help improve the ability of the pediatric field to come to terms with the complexities of the treatment and prevention of family violence (a problem with more dimensions than the purely medical). Thus, training efforts were addressed both to senior physicians who could, through their influence, enhance the "respectability" and value of a multidisciplinary approach to family violence, and to junior physicians who could develop enlightened perspectives and particular kinds of interpersonal skills before becoming locked into the narrower perspectives that characterize many specialty areas.

As the training program evolved, several approaches were used in the teaching sessions on family violence. During the first year of the program, an effort was made to get project staff included on the roster of every medical specialty's in-service teaching schedule, as well as the hospital's medical grand rounds and postgraduate rounds. Richard Gelles, the first postdoctoral fellow on the training grant, was enlisted in this effort. Dr. Gelles is a sociologist who already had established a national reputation for research in the area of family violence before he became a social science fellow on the training grant. In addition to publishing several books, chapters, and articles on family violence, he had collaborated with Straus and Steinmetz on the major study of family violence discussed in chapter 3 and published in the book *Behind Closed Doors: Violence in the American Family* (Straus, Gelles, and Steinmetz 1980).

A second approach to in-service education, case-focused teaching sessions, was used whenever a particularly difficult or upsetting case appeared on one of the hospital's medical or surgical services. These might include cases where serious disagreement occurred among medical and social service staff as to whether the child was at risk or whether the case should be referred to the Trauma X team. For example, when a child was diagnosed as having subdural hematomas of unclear etiology, the physician focusing narrowly on the symptom might insist on an accidental explanation, while the social worker and nursing staff might be convinced that social factors placed the child at great risk, even if the etiology was unclear. Such disagreements have serious implications, because if physicians in the emergency room miss a case of inflicted violence—for example, because of a missing medical record or a failure to ask the right question—the child may return later with more serious injuries. Other types of upsetting cases included those involving attempted or completed murder, which aroused strong emotions in all involved. In these situations, an attempt was made to set up a case-focused teaching conference, led either by Trauma X staff or, better yet, by the chief resident or chief of service in the division to which the child had been admitted. At these sessions, the course of case management would be reviewed, with focus on psychological and social data as well as on the medical data. In each case, an attempt was made to understand the etiology and plan an intervention; however, it was not possible in all cases to come to closure on whether the injury was inflicted or not.

A third approach to in-service teaching was carried out within disciplinary groups and was facilitated by the introduction of pediatric fellows into the training program. In this approach, pediatric fellows used case consultation with members of their own discipline as an educational vehicle, *whether such consultation was solicited or not.* This approach was found to be most useful when a sharp split or tension arose among staff members on how to manage a case.

Over the three years of the training program, the Trauma X faculty members and fellows conducted a total of 150 in-service teaching sessions within the hospital. They taught at almost every disciplinary and specialty in-service seminar. Reactions were positive, and relations between the Trauma X team and the hospital staff improved. The Trauma X team began to be consulted regularly by physicians from medical units who had previously been reluctant to deal directly with issues related to family violence. Although difficult cases continue to split staff in decision making, procedures have been established to address these splits and to facilitate collaboration.

5
The Model Hospital-based Training Program on Family Violence

O btaining federal grant support was very useful both in achieving the expanded level of in service education described in chapter 4 and in instituting two new components: a Family Violence Seminar and a fellowship program for pediatricians and behavioral and social scientists. Underlying all training program activities was a common set of goals, including heightening the professional awareness of the content and complexity of social problems associated with family violence, expanding the repertory of conceptual and practical tools of practitioners, promoting interdisciplinary communication and collaboration, and stimulating critical scrutiny of present knowledge and practice. It was hoped that exposure to new theories and methods would prompt participants to rethink and redirect professional commitments.

Training in the project focused on professional concepts and skills; however, components of the project, especially the weekly Family Violence Seminar, were also conceived as laboratories for investigating the basis for current beliefs and practices concerning family violence. One of the goals was the generation of a state-of-the-art training curriculum for guiding future research and practice. In other words, we hoped to develop an improved training model on family violence and, out of this, a curriculum that could assist future clinical management at Children's Hospital and other hospital facilities.

The Family Violence Seminar

The Family Violence Seminar was a key component of the training program, providing a weekly forum for presentations on family violence by researchers, policymakers, and clinicians. The seminar met every Tuesday morning for an hour and a half, with an average weekly attendance of twenty-five participants representing all professional groups at the hospital, as well as external health, mental health, and social service agencies and academic institutions. A core group of participants attended regularly while many others came periodically. Speakers were invited from within and outside the hospital and from academic, government, and clinical settings to share current research, issues in public policy, and innovations or expertise in clinical practice with the participants.

The Family Violence Seminar was designed to meet a number of goals identified by those hospital clinicians who were most involved in practice with victims of family violence and who had formulated the proposal for the training program. These goals included the following:

> Updating knowledge based on research, policy, and practice in the area of child maltreatment and family violence
>
> Providing a forum for discussion among clinicians of different disciplines and among clinicians and researchers
>
> Providing an opportunity for critical examination of the assumptions and concepts guiding clinical practice
>
> Considering current views on the etiology of family violence and sexual abuse, and the implications of these theories for practice
>
> Generating new conceptual models to guide the investigation of issues in family violence

An additional goal specific to the training program was to develop a curriculum on family violence useful to other professionals in the field. To this end, all seminars were taped. The onset of the training program provided a budget to free some of the project codirector's time to organize the seminar and to offer a modest honorarium for speakers.

To institute the Family Violence Seminar, an initial planning session was devoted to determining who the participants should be. A major goal of the seminar was to foster communication and better mutual understanding among those in the disciplines involved with child abuse cases in the hospital: nurses, social workers, pediatricians, psychiatrists, and psychologists. While social service and nursing staff had already expressed interest in attending the seminar, much thought had to be given to attracting pediatric staff who saw issues of family violence as generally outside their domain. Notices were placed in the weekly schedule of medical teaching events. Chiefs of services were contacted by phone to inform them about and invite them to the seminar. Much consideration was accorded the selection of speakers who might appeal most to the medical staff. Yet, overall, these efforts failed to attract much participation from the medical staff. The pediatricians who attended were those most intimately involved with the Trauma X team or already quite interested in the problem of family violence. Several pediatricians in ambulatory services attended occasionally, and one community pediatrician attended regularly for the first year of the program.

With social workers, nurses, and psychologists, the opposite problem was anticipated: so many would want to attend that the seminar would become too large to foster the kind of discussion desired. After much discussion, all social workers were invited to attend the seminar. The nurse on the project spoke with the head of nursing at the hospital regarding the project, and she assigned three nurses to attend the seminar. Selected psychologists and psychiatrists at the hospital and an affiliated child guidance clinic were also invited. Chiefs of all disciplines were invited. In addition, several social service agencies such as Parents' and Children's Services and the Department of Public Welfare were contacted to see whether they would like to send one or two representatives. Several local behavioral and social scientists involved in research on families were notified. In all, a total of eighty people were invited to attend the seminar, and there was an announcement in the medical area newsletter. Of this group, sixty-one attended at least one seminar, and a core group of twenty-five attended at least half of the seminars in the first year. The group composition, by discipline, was remarkably similar for all three years of the program, though many of the individual participants changed.

Over time, as word of the seminar spread, other members of the hospital community as well as representatives from outside agencies and universities asked if they might attend, and they were invited. Frequently, speakers invited for one meeting asked if they might become regular group members as well. Ultimately, representatives joined the seminar from a wide range of outside programs and projects, including an innovative family therapy outreach project from a mental health center funded by the state protective service agency; a counseling service for men who are violent toward their wives; several research projects, including a longitudinal study of the effects of abuse on children and a historical research project on sexual and family violence; a private child advocacy foundation; and the New England Resource Center for Protective Services.

The seminar went through some evolution in format during the first year. That period was considered experimental, and participants were urged to reflect critically on the seminar content and process in questionnaire evaluation and in several open discussion sessions. The first format used was that of the colloquium. Invited speakers gave presentations for as long as they wished, although they were advised to leave time for discussion. Weekly topics were varied and far-ranging. For example, one week the project codirector, a hospital attorney spoke on family violence and criminal law; the next week Richard Gelles, a sociologist and program fellow, presented the results of a national survey on family violence. These speakers were followed by a presentation on violence and children's television. Speakers in the first half of the first year were drawn mainly from the Boston area, and they focused on current research issues in family violence and sexual abuse, with occasional speakers on clinical or public policy issues.

In a questionnaire evaluation midway through the first year, the seminars were rated very positively, on the whole. However, two strong recommendations were made: (1) to provide more discussion time, and (2) to address clinical issues and applications for all the topics presented, even when the presenters focused only on research. These recommendations were followed. In the second and third years of the program, the seminars were organized into a modular format in which selected topics were considered during three presentations and one full session for discussion. This format provided more continuity and an opportunity to reflect on and integrate diverse approaches to the same issue.

The evolution of a group sense occurred slowly over the first year among the regular seminar attendees. It was not an easy process, however. Discussions were often competitive and conflict-ridden. Many members were silent and felt undervalued, in contrast to the "higher status" participants who dominated the floor. A discussion session devoted to the seminar process itself was helpful in bringing silent participants into the discussion and in raising group consciousness. Subsequent discussion sessions, however, though involving more members, continued to be conflictual. Frustration built up as participants felt that training program personnel were simply reflecting on the issues involved in the etiology of family problems, but were not really doing anything about them, or anything to improve the hospital practice with such cases. At one session set to discuss courses of possible action, the focus of the discussion was racism in the hospital structure and the responsibility of the seminar group to address this problem. The group was very divided as to what action to take. A newcomer to the seminar, who attended because of her interest in forming a group to study racism as it operated in the hospital, was criticized by two of the seminar participants for having an unworkable idea. The group was unable to agree on any unified goal, feelings ran high, and disciplinary lines often identified factions.

Nevertheless, all the participants continued to attend the seminar, and more and more became actively involved in expressing their views. By the end of the year, a regularly attending core group made up of members of all disciplines had emerged, expressing a commitment to attend the seminars the following year and an active interest in helping to plan and structure the next year's agenda.

As the seminar continued in the second year, a sense of a cohesive group, reflecting the contributions of all members, emerged. Discussions often reached an open and personal level as members talked about their own feelings, values, and experiences in such areas as sex roles, victimization, and race relations. The themes of sex roles, inequality, and aggression were prominent in discussions through much of the year, relating to presentations on sexual victimization of children, spouse abuse, and media exploitations of women. Discussions often led to consideration of the implications of these issues for relations among hospital professionals, or between professionals and patients. Although at times discussions of personal experiences related to gender or ethnic status became divisive, the overall effect was one of increasing cohesion and willingness to explore feelings and values.

Over time, whether the speaker was a researcher or clinician seemed to become less important. Research findings and ideas were freely discussed and criticized by clinicians, and applications to practice were suggested. Clinicians' presentations were discussed with great interest by researchers, who often were able to introduce relevant research findings that threw light on the clinical experience. The gap originally experienced between the two camps was bridged by a mutual interest in and respect for the others' work. In fact, many a participant remarked, "It doesn't really matter who speaks, or what they say, the discussion is the best part of the seminar."

The seminar was a meeting place for diverse individuals from diverse settings offering different perspectives on the problems of child maltreatment and family violence. As such, it served both intellectual and interpersonal functions. On an evaluation questionnaire, *all* respondents noted that their knowledge had been expanded through the seminar, and many called it a very stimulating part of their week. Academics and clinicians alike indicated that they looked forward to Tuesday mornings, as much to the exchange of perspectives in the discussion as to the presentation itself. Clinicians welcomed the opportunity to step back from their busy, at times overwhelming, caseload to reflect on and learn from a more abstract analysis of factors contributing to family problems. Researchers praised the unique opportunity to hear from clinicians working with families, and to learn from case material something about the clinical issues and frustrations in work with disabled families.

Many clinicians mentioned that their practice with families was affected by the seminar. Some reported an increased awareness of their personal biases and the assumptions they drew upon reaching conclusions about families. Many indicated an increased sympathy and empathy for all members of the family system, victim and perpetrator alike. Other clinicians became more critical of current clinical and protective interventions with families, and reported more ambivalence about what to do and more powerlessness to effect change. A number of clinicians, including members of the Trauma X team, indicated that their general approach to cases remained the same but that a stronger foundation of knowledge backed up what had previously been gut reactions. These clinicians reported increased confidence in their work and a growing tendency to advocate strongly for families and related policies.

In discussions of cases at the weekly Trauma X update meeting, which immediately followed the seminar, questions and comments frequently stemmed directly from the previous seminar. For example, following a presentation on the family system in cases of maltreatment, the usual emphasis on the mother's role was increasingly replaced by such questions as "What about the father?" and "What do we know about the rest of the family?" Seminars on minority families and economic and cultural factors in child abuse directly affected case discussions as well.

The seminar also stimulated other intellectual and training efforts for the participants. A participating lawyer organized an all-day workshop on family violence for juvenile court judges. A participating psychologist was prompted to finish and present a paper on power relations in violent families. On the basis of the success of the first year of the seminar, the Trauma X team organized a two-day workshop for state protective service workers.

The seminar also served an important interpersonal function. It allowed clinicians, who worked together in a very pressure- and crisis-oriented atmosphere, an opportunity to get to know one another in a less stressful setting. The developing sense of openness, respect, and cohesiveness among the participants affected overall working relationships.

Trauma X team members found that relationships with social workers and nurses attending the seminar developed new depth and respect. A firmer footing was established around difficult cases. Working relationships improved, and consultation became easier.

Fellows were frequently consulted by other seminar participants for advice on a research project, or for information regarding a teaching session. Hospital clinicians got to know and hear from representatives of the state protective service system, and greater respect, understanding, and cooperation ensued, as well as exchanges of practical information on particular cases.

Providing the opportunity for professionals to come together to learn and to talk to each other over time was the key element of the seminar. This program element was crucial. It had its difficult and conflict-filled moments, however, and, disappointingly, few pediatricians got involved. Persuading pediatricians to take time out from their busy medical schedules to learn more about family violence, particularly its psychosocial aspects, is likely to challenge organizers of training programs in other settings as well. Still, the effort to involve physicians is worthwhile; those pediatricians who did participate found it enormously helpful.

The Journal Group

Toward the end of the first year of the training program, an interdisciplinary journal group evolved. The purpose of this group was to review current theoretical and empiricial work in the area of family violence and to design and conduct empirical studies. The fellows were actively involved in research and writing efforts during their traineeship, and each developed papers that were presented at professional meetings and/or published. The journal group provided a congenial and helpful forum for the development of these projects and for trial runs on the papers presented. We would recommend this structure to practitioners in other clinical settings as a valuable format for interdisciplinary collaboration.

Fellowship Program

Postdoctoral fellowships were a component of the family violence training program which greatly facilitated the bridging of research and practice in the area of family violence. The fellowships were available to established behavioral and social scientists in the fields of psychology and sociology and to pediatricians with an interest in academic pediatrics and research. Although most settings are not able to provide federally supported fellowships to individuals at the postdoctoral level, the goals of our program and the experiences of our fellows are relevant to a variety of alternative approaches (for example, unpaid predoctoral traineeships) designed to bring researchers and practitioners together.

Bridging Research and Practice

Although the Family Violence Training Program was a clinical training program, its purpose was not to make clinicians out of social scientists but to improve the handling of family violence in medical settings by reducing the gap between research and practice. It was hoped that researchers and practitioners working together in a clinical setting would share their knowledge, insights, and perspectives in a way that would benefit everybody concerned with family violence. The training program provided a number of opportunities and structures for interchanges between researchers and practitioners, many of which took place specifically around concrete clinical cases.

The general goal of the fellowship program was to provide advanced training in the area of child maltreatment and family violence in a hospital setting and to foster careers in research on these problems. For pediatric fellows, a more specific goal was to provide intensive clinical exposure to interdisciplinary case evaluation and management as well as exposure to research knowledge and skills in the area of family violence and child maltreatment. For academic fellows already versed in research knowledge and skills, it was hoped that exposure to a clinical setting would promote clinical research on problems of family violence.

Two additional goals of the fellowship program were (1) to provide the wider hospital community with the research knowledge and conceptual skills of the academic fellows through informal consultation, collaboration, and teaching; and (2) to provide the pediatric staff with role model consultants and peers through the pediatric fellows.

To further these goals, a core set of training activities was planned for all fellows. These activities included the following:

Participation as presenters and discussants in the Family Violence Seminar

Participation in the Trauma X team update meetings, case conferences, and rounds—either as observers (academic fellows) or as participating clinicians (pediatric fellows)

Participation as observers and clinicians in the Family Development Clinic—as observers and supervised interviewers (academic fellows) or as principal clinicians (pediatricians)

Participation as presenters and discussants at other teaching activities within the hospital

After the second year, participation in a research-oriented journal group

Other training options included participation in the hospital's Child Development Program, Early Childhood Clinic, sexual abuse team, Department of Psychiatry seminar and rounds, and the failure-to-thrive team.

Introducing a training program on family violence requires preparation for dealing with the strong emotional impact of these cases. Our fellows provide, in their own words, clear indications of the kinds of reactions that program supervisors must be prepared to address. For example, in a pediatric hospital, cases of possible maltreatment often differ in their impact on the professional involved with them. In some weeks, cases of possible neglect or nonorganic failure to thrive can come to seem almost routine, even to the novice social science fellow. In other weeks, every case seems to arouse rage or despair. Some children undergoing prolonged hospitalization continue to have heart-rending impact through weeks and weeks of evaluation and review.

There are cases I came into contact with at Trauma X meetings that I will never forget as long as I live. I can still remember one of the first cases I heard about in Trauma X that continued over weeks and weeks. I remember those cases for the horror of what had happened to the kids and also for the difficulty there was in doing anything to help them.

Direct involvement of behavioral and social science fellows in the provision of psychotherapy (through the Department of Psychiatry) revealed no magical solution here either. Even when diagnoses had been made and agreed upon, and a course of psychotherapy had been recommended and undertaken, progress could be slow and elusive. Social science fellows who had assumed they could have a direct and immediate positive effect on families often brought feelings of frustration to their supervisors in psychiatry as well as to their mentors on the training program faculty.

> I never anticipated the level of involvement, of emotional and psychological involvement, with families. I guess I was expecting a small, discrete set of issues that we could address doing diagnostics or in clinics or through psychotherapy that could resolve within a few sessions. I never anticipated the ongoing nature, the kind of pile-up you get, so that just when you think you are making progress in one area, the dike breaks in another area. Yes, you are making progress but it is not like the nice linear progress I was expecting.

Bringing social scientists into a pediatric hospital meant dealing not only with their feelings about cases of family violence but also with their feelings about the cumbersome and imperfect process involved in diagnosing and treating such cases. Indeed, having a clinical training program in family violence meant having outsiders present as witnesses to all the problems of interdisciplinary cooperation and all the effects of the gap between research and practice—and again, dealing with the feelings and reactions of both the fellows and the hospital staff as a result of this addition.

For the pediatric fellows, involvement with Trauma X cases was of a more direct, medical nature, and it often provided a rather different set of experiences. For one of the pediatric fellows, working with the Trauma X team offered a much more positive experience than he had had earlier in his training.

> I don't think, strictly speaking, that we were working in isolation in my previous experience as a resident—there was usually

a social worker involved and we did report to the Bureau of Child Welfare—but the perception was that you were alone dealing with the anxieties and doubts that the different cases raise. Whereas here, the perception was one of close working relationships and of support—and that everybody was dealing with the same emotional burden and you had the opportunity to talk about it.

The presence of the fellows, and their expressions of thoughts and feelings concerning the processes they were observing, unavoidably—and perhaps usefully—had an impact on the medical and social service staff committed to dealing with cases of family violence. Professionals intending to develop family violence programs at other institutions should be prepared to deal with the fact that providing training to outsiders—especially, perhaps, if they are researchers—will affect all concerned.

Whatever disillusionments may have been connected with some aspects of the clinical experiences to which the fellows were exposed, they were also seen as valuable. Social science and clinical fellows alike found that their experience within the clinical services enriched their perspectives.

The experiences that had the most profound impact on me were the Family Development Clinic and the individual therapeutic and diagnostic work, where I had the opportunity in a one-to-one relationship to apply whatever research was applicable. It wasn't a static process where one takes research and applies it. It was back and forth and all the time. Clinical work opened up new ideas for interpreting research findings, and research findings were applied to clinical work with various degrees of success.

It's useful for practitioners to have researchers to tell them when they're pinning their diagnosis on a fallacious assertion. I remember a classic example where the clinician decided a fractured skull wasn't due to child abuse because it was administered by a sibling. I asked, "Well, gee, where do you think the sibling learned that kind of behavior?" A whole new discussion ensued with the social service people saying, "The house wasn't a mess. There couldn't be any abuse or neglect." I told them one has nothing to do with the other. On the other hand, the researchers say, "This is clearly a case of such and such," and the clinicians say, "We can't do a darn thing about that. Come up with something useful."

I think this is an ideal setting because the program brings together people of a research background with people of a clinical background around the same data—the same families in the clinic. Certainly, in my own development, the program helped me establish research questions that I thought were important and supplied me with the beginnings of the research tools to attack those questions.

I think I have a more profound appreciation, for example, of childhood accidents. Looking back, probably stemming from a rather optimistic view of human nature, I really used to have the perspective that accidents were much more random. Now I'd want to explore more deeply what led up to an accident. In the past, as a physician confronted by an accident, if supplied with a plausible explanation, I think I would have treated it lightly. Now I feel that in certain instances I would see the accident as pointing to stress, for example, or some family dysfunction. And I'd probe more deeply to assess whether or not there were family issues manifesting in those accidents and needing to be addressed.

There was a fair amount of discussion about some difficult clinical issues and I really enjoyed that. As a small bonus package to a pediatrician, it was of value to be exposed to the area of handicapped children and their treatment. It was very helpful to have the opportunity of working in a multidisciplinary group and to see firsthand what are the common, profound dilemmas that lead to research.

I think clinical training should be part of every psychologist's training. It's too easy to be an armchair psychologist, to elaborate your theories and design your studies in the abstract, without knowing, for example, what it feels like to be a clinician dealing with a case. If researchers are going to talk to clinicians, they have to know what it feels like to work with a child who was beaten up. And if researchers are going to write in a way that is useful for anybody besides journal editors and other professionals—and I think it's their responsibility to do so—then it helps to have some ground-level experience. My experience in talking with mothers and observing mothers and kids interacting behind the one-way mirror in the Family Development Clinic and seeing how cases got dealt with in Trauma X did that for me, made me want to write for a broad audience. For a basic researcher and academician, that kind of real-life experience makes you understand the realities you're dealing with, how difficult and complex it is to make the world a better place.

As a researcher, I originally conceptualized family violence in terms of battering—a very narrow kind of conceptualization. Working with the Trauma Team as well as in some of my clinical experiences, I came in contact with a variety of cases that weren't violent in a narrow interpretation of inflicted injury. I can think of a specific case where a child was injured by an automobile door. Irrespective of whether that injury was consistent with the explanation, there were a whole host of other family dynamics which led the clinicians to view this family as a family in trouble and at risk. In terms of the narrow definition of battering with which I came, that child was not battered, but he certainly was a victim of one form of maltreatment.

Issues in Clinical Training

The clinical component of the Family Violence Training Program, like the other components, was dynamic, not static. It evolved over time and in response to the expressed needs and concerns of the fellows. In this section, we review the major issues raised by the fellows concerning their clinical training and the changes made in this component of the training program to deal with those issues. Again, both the issues raised and the responses made are relevant to all clinical settings that recognize the need to undertake training on family violence.

Orientation

The fellows, even those with previous clinical experience, expressed a need for orientation to and debriefing after clinical case presentations and clinical observations. No one felt prepared for the emotional onslaught that accompanied hearing about and dealing with case after case of family violence and severe deprivation in the lives of children and their parents. In the Family Development Clinic, academic fellows asked for some explication and discussion of the clinical processes they were observing, such as interviews by psychiatrists and social workers, and assessments by nurses and clinical psychologists. Pediatric fellows requested close supervision on cases with which they were involved, feeling that their previous training had not sufficiently prepared them for parent and family interviewing, negotiating with social service and judicial personnel, or testifying in court. In addition, fellows were eager to learn about hospital procedures and politics likely to affect the management of family violence cases.

A number of steps were taken to respond to trainee requests for expanded supervision and enlightenment. Beginning in the second year of the program, a series of individual orientation meetings was arranged for the pediatric fellows with Ms. Betty Singer, the Trauma X chairperson. In addition, all fellows were assigned an adviser-mentor from the program faculty to facilitate their entry into the training program and hospital, and to provide an orientation and opportunity for discussion of clinical observations and experiences. Advisors and fellows attempted to meet once a week or biweekly. Regular monthly meetings for all fellows were scheduled with the project evaluator to review training activities and issues. Finally, in the third year of the program, an hour was arranged for case discussion following Family Development Clinic appointments on Thursday afternoons. This time was used to discuss the cases seen that afternoon and to generate research questions relevant to the clinical process—for example, issues related to the assessment tools used in studying family interaction.

Association with Psychiatry Department

Some of the social science fellows elected to obtain supervised psychotherapy experience from the hospital's Department of Psychiatry and expressed a need for a closer tie-in between the department and the training program. The fellows desired more discussion of the experience within Psychiatry than was possible during regular supervision on cases. Psychiatry department supervisors tended to assume that the behavioral and social science fellows were well-versed in psychiatric concepts and perspectives. Jargon was often confusing. Both supervisors and fellows sought to clarify the purpose of this training experience.

To facilitate the fellows' integration of this experience, Dr. Carolyn Newberger, a psychologist on the program faculty, took on two additional responsibilities in the third year of the project: (1) supervision of the fellows in diagnostic evaluations and psychotherapy, and (2) leadership of a seminar on psychiatric perspectives where issues related to the connections between research and practice were discussed with the fellows.

Clearly, both the pediatric and social science fellows found their training year to be an enlightening and enriching experience—although they generally did not believe that either the clinical or other components of the training program had radically altered their perspectives on family violence. The absence of radical changes in perspectives is not surprising. Application and selection procedures in a clinical training program such as ours are likely to ensure a certain degree of open-mindedness and freedom from a blaming-the-victim mentality in its trainees. These were precisely the attitudes that were fostered within the training program, along with, of course, both scientific objectivity and clinical sensitivity. Moreover, all the fellows came into the program with a desire somehow to build on their own interests and skills in ways that would be helpful to families and to the eventual alleviation of family violence. In all cases, the program proved consistent with and supportive of these goals.

As a result of their experiences in the clinical services, reality was broadened for practitioners and social scientists alike. The clinicians developed new sets of cognitive lenses through which to view troubled families. The social scientists were brought much closer to real-world problems than had been possible in their university settings. Both practitioners and social scientists questioned some of their old answers and began formulating new questions about families. Together, social scientists and practitioners generated research questions, giving rise to a substantial number of investigations, some of which have been completed and some of which are still under way. Moreover, all the fellows are likely to be involved in teaching/training activities for the rest of their professional lives, and all of them believe that these activities have been influenced by their participation in the training program.

6
Professional Roles in the Service and Training Program in Family Violence

The Multidisciplinary Case Conference

Family violence services began at Children's Hospital at a time when the problems of child abuse, child sexual abuse, and family violence were only dimly perceived and were often ignored within the medical services. When the Trauma X consultation unit was formed in 1970, communication within the principal human service disciplines was inadequate, and the isolation of the hospital from community service agencies was very evident. The first task was to convene a weekly multidisciplinary case conference involving representatives from the hospital, the public social welfare agency mandated by law to receive child abuse case reports, and two private child welfare agencies with special competencies in the child protection area.

The lessons learned from this experience guided the subsequent development of written hospital guidelines for child abuse case management. These guidelines stipulated particular roles for individual members and for the consultation unit as a whole. A more in-depth discussion of issues of case management can be found in appendix C. The following six lessons learned from the multidisciplinary conference are worthy of attention in all medical facilities concerned with family violence:

1. The social work discipline must be central, both in the administrative locus of the consultative unit and in the leadership

of the team. We found that placing the program under the aegis of the hospital's general administration, rather than a particular medical department, gave social work the needed standing. Conferences led by physicians, psychiatrists, and lawyers, no matter how sensitive these persons were to the process or how informed about the issues, often tended to intimidate social workers from the hospital as well as from other agencies. Despite their traditionally lower status, social workers and nurses are most often able to discern and pinpoint the family dimensions of violence or of sexual abuse. Moreover, these professionals have firsthand access to the information on adults, children, and family relationships on which important diagnostic and custody judgments and choices are made. Consequently, conferences are most successful in encouraging a full sense of participation when chaired by a social worker. Moreover, consensus appears to evolve more easily and conflict seems to be tolerated more readily when the chair is a social worker. In medical and legal institutions, the important power prerogatives are often held, if not zealously guarded, by men. Giving social workers and nurses, who traditionally have been women, a visible leadership and decision-making role conveys to various colleagues the message that these are professionals deserving respect and esteen.

2. *Issues of turf and control are best approached through discussion and patience, not through promulgation of rules, procedures, and rigid stipulation of roles.* Such is the nature of medical specialties. In our hospital, for example, the task of empowering the nursing and social service professionals was initially attempted by drafting edicts and guidelines; ultimately, however, success came through steady and consistent consultation and teaching. That is, only gradually was it possible to persuade certain of the specialty medical and surgical services to relinquish elements of their total control over the patient. Now, after fourteen years of in-service teaching conferences and efforts to give higher visibility and respect to the work of social workers and nurses, these professionals can, without the orders or permission of physicians, make direct contact with the consultation team. Occasional carping on the part of certain of the older members of the physician staff remains, but the principle is generally accepted.

Establishing links between individual members of the consultation team and counterparts on each of the specialty services was a particularly useful way to gain respect for a consultation group that took a very different approach to patients and their families than had been traditional in a medical setting. Attitudes of support, appreciation, and professionalism were of greater value than the prevalent postures of competition and struggle. Fostering human values in a personal approach to one's colleagues appealed to all participants.

3. *The best decision making derives from discussions where conflict is permitted and different professionals' perspectives can be expressed.* Often, difficult judgments must be based on limited and subjective information. Good decisions require time for sorting out information from inferences and for defining the reliability, validity, and meaning of the information. The tendency on the part of the professionals in medicine, psychiatry, nursing, and social work—based on their professional training and socialization—is to derive pathologic or illness formulations from information about families. An opportunity for open expression of views about strength and health, as well as an understanding of different cultural values and their manifestations in family life, permits development of a better ability to conceptualize and to acknowledge strength as well as pathology or problems. With this process goes a certain amount of ambiguity and conflict, but the decisions that emerge may be more humane and conducive to better health in children.

4. *Unless issues of class and cultural bias are brought forth explicitly in consultations and case conferences, decisions will, however unintentionally, be influenced by such biases.* We have learned to identify explicitly the socioeconomic status of the family, their culture, ethnicity, and race, and to note specifically the need to consider the family information with respect to the cultural context. Having a mix of professionals from various backgrounds assists enormously in controlling a propensity toward culture-bound value judgments.

5. *The natural tendency for professionals faced with a difficult decision is to call for additional information.* This is especially true if the family is middle class or affluent, because professionals

are frequently reluctant, when a family is similar to their own, to derive diagnoses carrying a negative value judgment. One can hear professionals saying essentially, "Why, they're such a nice, well-to-do family. They couldn't be abusing their child. If we get more information it will become clear that those injuries couldn't be due to abuse." In actuality, preliminary information is often sufficient for a diagnosis of maltreatment, and indeed, the information would be acknowledged as sufficient if the family were poor or otherwise disadvantaged. What is typically needed in such situations is not more information about the family, not another consultation, but a coming to grips with the reality that child maltreatment can take place even in nice, professional families just like the folks next door.

It is valuable to have available, within the interdisciplinary case team, professionals representing the range of disciplines from which consultations are likely to be called. For example, often the only agreement about a family violence case is that a psychiatric consultation is needed. The presence of a psychiatrist may help to inform the participants that although psychodiagnostic information can sometimes be very useful, it is not likely to provide solutions in this particular case. Similarly, although the option of leaving a difficult judgment to a court may appear to be very attractive, having a lawyer on the consultation team may help the medical personnel understand the limits of the adversary process and the capriciousness of many of its judgments. It may be that only a lawyer can convince physicians and social workers that "a recommendation to let the courts figure it out" is not a viable way of extricating oneself and one's colleagues from a difficult decision-making situation.

6. *Visiting clinical and social science professionals both help and hinder the case consultation process.* On the one hand, nothing matches the new, fresh perspective of an informed visitor. In our experience with consultations on family violence, the occasional visiting scholar or clinician was often able to voice questions or to present corroborative information in such a way as to prompt the clinicians to think through the data differently. For example, in a case involving both spouse and child abuse, where it appeared that the juvenile court was going to force the wife to choose between

a depressed husband and a severely beaten two-year-old, a visiting sociologist noted that this forced choice might create the kind of double bind seen often in murder-suicides. That is, murder-suicides can occur in circumstances where an individual believes that he or she has no alternative except to choose between two equally horrifying sets of circumstances. Thus, the mother in this case may feel so conflicted that she might end up killing her child, then herself. This comment stimulated a reanalysis of the family relationships at the level of the family, as well as the parent-child dyad.

On the other hand, visitors can also have a negative effect on the group dynamics of clinical communication and formulation. Often a clinician may try to play to or show off for a visitor, or bend over backwards to make a teaching point, or take time to explain courteously what is going on. His or her colleagues may seethe with impatience or suppressed laughter at such antics, and the respectful and open communication that is so essential to sound practice may be compromised.

Disciplinary Roles

The task of assembling the proposal for the training grant led in 1978 to a discussion of the roles that each of the disciplines might play in the work of training. With the above lessons held in view, consensus was reached on the particular array of responsibilities to be met by the professionals involved in the training of the fellows. The roles of these professionals within the family violence service and training program are described next.

Social Workers

Social workers at Children's Hospital are responsible for evaluating interactions among family members, forming relationships with other hospital programs and community agencies that will be a foundation for successful external referrals for service, and making arrangements for these referrals. Social workers are available in the emergency clinic on a twenty-four-hour basis. The family violence program had available to it three principal social workers:

the chief of the social service department, the head of its community services division (who also chaired the child abuse consultation team), and the social worker for the outpatient Family Development Clinic, where family violence–related consultations take place (Newberger and McAnulty 1976).

As part of the training program, all fellows were expected to attend clinical conferences chaired by social workers and dealing with cases of family violence. The social worker chairperson or another social worker was asked to spend an hour a week debriefing each postdoctoral fellow and discussing the issues at hand. In practice, this arrangment worked for some fellows but not for others. Often the press of the social worker's clinical responsibilities reduced the debriefing hour at both ends. Though some fellows thought they received enough input despite the demands on their assigned mentor's schedule, other fellows were frustrated at the lack of time to help them work through the thoughts and feelings that accompanied their exposure to family violence cases. The ratio of fellows to social workers increased over the life of the project, during which (and partly as a consequence of which) the visibility of the issues and the number of case consultation requests climbed substantially.

Nurses

A pediatric nurse practitioner whose half-time hospital appointment included assignments to the child abuse consultation unit and Family Development Clinic was available as a faculty member in the training program. Her tasks in the hospital included serving as a liaison with the nurses both in administration and on the clinical services. In this capacity, she was responsible for arranging teaching conferences, in which the fellows were invited on occasion to participate. For the fellows, she served as a strong and secure leader in her profession. Her contacts with the fellows were continuous and informal. Only rarely were formal appointments needed to sustain her input into the fellows' training. Much of her own work was in the context of the Family Development Clinic, where the one-way mirror is used in family evaluations for the dual purposes of teaching and of restricting the number of personnel in the examining room with the family. Frequently, she was the clinician observed through the mirror; at other times she participated as an observer, giving information and consultation to the fellows as the work with the family went forward.

Pediatricians

The pediatricians associated with the training program included its director, the senior pediatrician on the interdisciplinary child abuse consultation unit, and the chief of the hospital's primary care program. Each physician worked in a context with considerable clinical exposure to family violence cases. These contexts proved useful to the fellows as a source of pertinent data and case material. Each pediatrician's responsibilities included serving as administrative liaison to the clinical and administrative departments with which the fellows had contacts. The pediatricians also represented the program to clinical department chiefs; on the rare occasions when conflicts involving a fellow emerged, the pediatricians acted to troubleshoot and negotiate a solution. Among the clinicians, the pediatricians seemed most interested in making contact with behavioral and social scientists to initiate research in the family violence area.

Lawyers

The hospital's attorney played a vital and unique role in the program. The treatment of family violence inevitably involves ethical and legal dilemmas (especially regarding confidentiality and informed consent) and brings the courts into play. In this context, the attorney interpreted the legal framework for professional action and guided decision making. His advice covered such situations as whether to file a child abuse report, whether and how to initiate a custody action on a child's behalf, how to file a spouse abuse petition, whether to retain a child in the hospital, and whether or how to inform a mother that her child, in state custody, had been murdered while in foster home care. The training program was fortunate to attract an attorney with a substantive interest in family violence, child custody, and interdisciplinary clinical work.

Psychologists and Psychiatrists

Opportunities were provided for fellows to conduct supervised diagnostic assessments of parents and children in the hospital's psychiatric outpatient department, and several fellows availed themselves of the chance to do psychotherapy under the aegis of the psychiatry department. Those who did become involved in providing psychotherapy participated in the pertinent weekly seminars in the psychiatry department; supervision of their clinical work was provided by two psychologists and one psychiatrist. The fellows brought to this work an orientation to theory and an energy that attracted the interest and support of the supervising professionals, all of whom reported that they learned enormously from the experience. One of the fellows, Dr. Richard Gelles, has reported at length on his clinical training experience in his paper "Applying Research on Family Violence to Clinical Practice" (1982).

The introduction of the training program added extra work for hospital clinical staff. Moreover, as a consequence of the fellows' lack of familiarity with some of the unwritten codes of behavior in medical environments, some conflicts occurred with the professionals identified as faculty in the program. Strong feelings are inevitable in the family violence area; these feelings occasionally energized discussions about the program and interactions with the fellows in troublesome ways. For example, behavioral and social science fellows were sometimes eager to share research knowledge relevant to a case being considered in a Trauma X meeting or case conference. When the day's schedule was already very heavy, such input sometimes seemed intrusive and unhelpful to the clinical staff, who wished the fellows would save their insights for some less busy occasion.

Because misunderstandings and hurt feelings could arise under such circumstances, it proved useful to have weekly meetings with the fellows, conducted by a psychologist, to help them process their experiences as individuals and as a group. Also important were the fellows' meetings with members of the identified clinical faculty. These meetings served to cement a sense of common purpose and to place in perspective personal and professional differences. The former always healed with time; the latter came increasingly to be understood as artifacts of the differing intellectual orientations of the clinical and research disciplines. People came to know and to respect one another as individuals, and to comprehend the different ways in which they look at the world.

7

Conclusions and Recommendations

The Interdisciplinary Team Approach

As we have seen, child abuse/neglect management at Children's Hospital is the responsibility of an interdisciplinary team consisting of a pediatrician, attorney, psychiatric social worker, psychologist, nurse, and occasional other consultants. Such a team structure has several advantages over individual management and decision making.

Advantages of Team Structure

Cases of family violence involve many specialties, each with differing and unique definitions of the situation presented. If, for example, a child enters the emergency ward with a fracture, the physician might determine whether the nature of the break indicates inflicted trauma; the social worker would interview the child's parents to evaluate their capacity to protect the child and to form a relationship that might serve as the basis for a program to prevent the injury from recurring; and the attorney might consider obtaining a restraining order to prevent removal of the child from the hospital prior to a full assessment. The primary rationale for an interdisciplinary team, then, is that many skills are required for effective task performance.

A team approach, moreover, has other functions or advantages specifically in regard to family violence. First, these problems stimulate strong emotional reactions in all of us; anger, sadness, and frustration are all too familiar. If group management exists, members can support one another and allay some of the personal distress inevitably associated with tragedy. Second, decision making in this area affects family welfare and the safety and health of children. A group can bear the consequences of its decisions more easily than can an individual who selects and lives with his or her recommendations alone. Third, family violence cases are complex and take much time and effort to resolve. A team is able to divide the labor to facilitate the outcomes. (See appendix C.)

Team Issues

Before any team can function effectively, a number of questions must be raised and certain group issues must be recognized:

1. *What are the norms of practice—that is, what are the expectations or rules that exist within the group?* In order for a team to perform well, consensus must exist about what rules apply to the group and to individual participants. For example, all members might agree that everyone should participate in decisions concerning the disposition of serious cases, but the levels of participation might differ according to the nature of the decision (whether it is primarily legal or involves medical diagnosis or social service assessment).

2. *What roles do individuals play, and how might these roles change over time?* After operating in an interdisciplinary setting for a period of time, participants become comfortable with the language and thought processes of each other's specialties. The pediatrician, for example, might venture a psychiatric assessment, or the social worker a legal analysis. This crossing of disciplines is usually done with the realization that turf is being violated; apologies are given ("I don't mean to get into your area . . ."), statements qualified ("I'm no lawyer, but . . ."), or immediate deference shown if the nonexpert statement is challenged by the authority. In this way, members feel sufficiently free to transcend their narrow roles but not so much as to threaten or question the capacity of their associates.

3. *What is the status and power structure within the team?* In a hospital setting, physicians usually have the greatest authority or influence; within teams it becomes possible—indeed, perhaps essential—to emphasize professional collegiality rather than hierarchy.

4. *How is social cohesion maintained?* In the interdisciplinary team, multiple divisions exist that can potentially disrupt unity and harm morale. These divisions include differing professional orientations and commitments; ideological variations; diverse interpersonal styles; and sex, race, and social class distinctions. Problem solving is sometimes limited by different professionals viewing the same data in different ways, and an inability across disciplines to understand the concepts and tools of other specializations. In considering a particular case of family violence, a sociologist analyzing the causes of abuse probably would look to the social context in which the behavior occurs—the strains or pressures that triggered aggression. A psychologist, on the other hand, might focus on the individual perpetrator. Examining past experiences as a predictor of present action, he or she might ask, "What kind of person would act in this way?" and might attempt to construct a psychological profile from developmental history and from attitudinal/behavioral data. To a psychologist, social context is often the circumstance precipitating violence rather than its primary cause; the violence, defined as endemic, may be considered inevitable, despite the chance stimulus that induced it. The social worker may find all such considerations too abstract and be much more concerned with helping family members cope with circumstances that appear overwhelming.

Suggestions on Team Functioning

Though what works at Children's Hospital may not generalize readily to other programs, the following suggestions on team functioning may prove helpful:

1. *Attempt to draft a written statement on team norms and practices.* At Children's, the team norms, for the most part, are

not codified; however, a handbook written by the group outlines the task(s) each participant is to perform. The handbook attempts to standardize decision making by indicating when various procedures are appropriate (for example, taking a trauma case to court). This handbook is considered important because it educates members and lessens arbitrariness; a latent function is the reduction of conflict. We attempt to use guidelines to avoid differences of opinion and to resolve those differences that do arise.

2. *Set aside a minimum of one meeting a week to discuss team functioning and organizational/personal issues.* Too often the pressure of caseloads and clinical decision making limits the group's ability to assess *group process.* Any team needs to devote time to itself and not simply to case management.

3. *Hold weekly update meetings with all team members.* At these meetings consider the medical/psychiatric data on *all* cases seen at the hospital since the last session. This sharing permits each member to know about every case and to ask for additional information or to provide an expert opinion. The group thus maintains itself as a group and takes advantage of the interdisciplinary skills of its members.

4. *Have each member participate in case decision making* according to the specific issues requiring decision. The pediatrician, for example, might examine a patient to determine whether injuries are accidental, a result of disease, or inflicted, while the lawyer might assess the medical record to determine whether the evidence is sufficient to meet a burden of proof requirement if the team urges removal of a child from biological parents and the initiation of court action.

5. *Attempt to reach a consensus* on important issues of case management—for example, whether a child abuse or neglect report should be filed with state protective services or a neglect (care and protection) petition initiated. If all participants agree with particular courses of action, then team division is less likely. If strong differences do occur, however, especially between the medical and social work perspectives, no action should be taken until efforts at resolution are made. Any remaining differences might be resolved by a respected and neutral third party, such as a hospital administrator.

6. *Accept, and indeed encourage, different opinions* on case management, as they often lead to more intelligent decisions. On the other hand, keep in mind the fact that if argument becomes

too intense or personal, team solidarity suffers. It is important, therefore, to consider social-emotional factors and the need for norms that allow team members to continue working with one another. Typical informal norms might include (*a*) maintaining equanimity in disagreement, (*b*) resolving disagreement through rational discussion, and (*c*) being supportive of one another (by showing solidarity). It is important to keep things cool and to maintain a sense of humor.

7. *Share power.* Despite the fact that in the larger society, and particularly in the hospital, a physician has greater authority and status than does a nurse or social worker, the team should operate under a norm of collegiality. This norm has several components: all disciplines are equally important in decision making; the quality and logic of a suggestion is more important than the status of the person offering it; and no person or role representative has the right to veto a recommendation acceptable to other group members. This norm increases individual assertiveness and the feeling that one may operate without fear of sanction—all of which leads to group morale, commitment, and cohesion. Task effectiveness is likewise enhanced. No single discipline has greater knowledge or insight into family violence management than the others; thus, no single discipline should be accorded weight merely because of what it is, as opposed to what it contributes.

One way to share power is to rotate the role of conference chairperson rather than having the same discussion leader at each meeting. This device, of course, might merely disguise the true power structure; however, if used properly, it can enhance team collegiality. It is also valuable if a physician takes the responsibility for acknowledging the importance of the nursing and social work perspectives and approaches rather than leaving it to members of those disciplines to assert their own value.

Institutional Issues and Team Functioning

In a medical center with a biomedical orientation and a deemphasis on child development, trauma teams may lack social and economic support. In this case, the team should fall within the jurisdiction of a hospital administrator who can act as its advocate. The team should also receive financial support from the institution rather than relying on grant monies or private contributions. Without financial backing, the professionals will not remain committed to the difficult work of case management; moreover, task quality will suffer because of a lack of secretaries, computers, or other facilitators.

Within the hospital setting, teams exhibit either a consultative or a directive mode of operation. In the consultative mode, members consult with other professionals who actually provide services to families. The team pediatrician, for example, may conduct a medical examination to determine whether fractures resemble inflicted injuries, but the house officer, after receiving input, maintains case control and makes decisions about abuse/neglect reporting and discharge. In the directive mode, the staff of the various hospital divisions transfer management responsibility to the abuse team, which provides services and assessment while also determining case disposition.

At Children's Hospital, though the formal procedure is consultative, actual team functioning may become directive. Certain staff members dislike child abuse cases and willingly surrender responsibility to the "experts." Others have a strong sense of turf and clearly indicate their desire for the trauma team to play a subordinate role. With the most serious cases of abuse/neglect, however, especially those that involve court petitions, the team becomes more directive even with those professionals who would otherwise wish for independence. If the lawyer, for example, believes that psychiatric evaluation of the parents would assist his or her presentation of a court petition, staff psychiatrists may be pressured to defer even when they see no clinical need for the evaluation.

Because of the confusion between consultative and directive orientations, questions often arise over which decisions should be made by the team and which should be made by other hospital staff. Questions also arise as to how authority and case control should be divided between staff and team. Team members expend much effort to avoid offending division staff and attempt, through sensitive persuasion, to get division staff to do what the team recommends.

Unfortunately, many hospital staffers do not like the trauma team or trauma cases. The team is seen as interfering or disruptive, for example, by considering social issues while physicians want merely to mend the broken bone and send the patient home. Abuse cases are complex, unpleasant, and demanding.

Group cohesion within the team is sometimes increased by this sense of being outsiders within the hospital community. Team members begin to believe that only they are concerned about the welfare of the total child and that legitimate needs of children and families are being slighted. Members may also fear that team expertise is going unrecognized or that lack of consultations will threaten team survival. Too much of a we/they orientation, however, only isolates the team from other colleagues and creates member alienation and burnout.

In our experience, family violence training program directors can contribute significantly to improved relationships between the trauma team and others by inviting staff to seminars and by finding behavioral and social scientists to teach on the unit. Such efforts give the trauma team credibility as a force that can attract talented professionals or preprofessionals who wish to learn from its members.

It is also important for the team members to maintain links to their own discipline—the nurse to nurses, the social worker to social workers. When problems arise within a particular discipline, the team professional in that discipline can attempt to resolve intergroup conflicts.

Guiding Principles

From our early experiences in developing a family violence service program, we established a set of principles to guide our Family Violence Training Program. Each of these principles was designed to address concrete problems in case management, to facilitate interdisciplinary cooperation, and to bring the relevant conceptual and empirical tools into effective operation in a hospital setting. These principles have withstood the test of time, and we recommend them to individuals in other settings who wish to address the problems raised by a desire to respond more effectively to family violence.

1. *Develop broader and more adequate conceptual perspectives for medical and other health practice.* Problems in clinical practice make it clear that more adequate intellectual tools are greatly needed in the family violence area. Health personnel need to be more aware of the complexity and many dimensions of the family violence problem, including the policy and functional implications of the diagnostic labels that they may apply in the course of such practice. Careful attention needs to be given by clinicians to the adequacy (or inadequacy) of concepts such as child abuse and child neglect as a basis for practice. Clinicians should be given an opportunity to consider whether emphasis in the family violence area should be directed solely at the specific illness of the patient or expanded to include the evaluation of the patient's needs within the family and social setting (Newberger, Newberger, and Richmond 1976).

2. *Promote greater cooperation among health and mental health professionals rendering clinical services.* Problems of family violence are interstitial in the sense that several different fields need to work together to provide effective treatment and service. In a case of child abuse or interspousal violence, a physician may treat the physical injury while a social worker obtains the family history and an attorney advises on the legal aspects. Unfortunately, because of specialized and narrow professional training, persons of different disciplines may not relate effectively to each other and to human needs in cases of family violence. Another factor to be considered is that the health workers who often seem best able to understand the familial and social contexts—psychologists, social workers, nurses—often have minimal access to the physicians and attorneys who make major decisions. Thus, means should be sought to lessen or eliminate such barriers to effective provision of health services.

3. *Increase sensitivity of health care providers to cultural, social, ethnic, and economic factors that have important implications for effective service.* Hospital clientele often come from ethnic, socioeconomic, and cultural groups different from those of the providers of health care. Such differences can make it difficult for health care personnel to develop rapport with persons needing assistance in the family violence area, or to understand and treat effectively the individual and social problems presented to them. Poor and/or minority persons are more readily labeled and

stigmatized as child abusers and wife beaters and their cases managed coercively (for example, with removal of the child from the family or notification of police) than are patients who are more affluent or influential (Newberger and Bourne 1978, Bourne and Newberger 1977).

4. *Promote more productive communication and collaboration among professionals in clinical practice and behavioral and social science research.* Ways need to be found to relate family violence research more effectively to clinical needs, and to use exposure to clinical practice as a means of sensitizing researchers to clinical concerns. Improved communication between the worlds of research and practice can assist greatly in developing improved conceptual and theoretical frameworks for practice, and in encouraging interdisciplinary research efforts and findings of practical value to clinical practice.

What steps can be taken to accomplish those goals in other settings, particularly settings that cannot offer postdoctoral fellowships to clinicians and academicians interested in family violence? Clearly, the financial constraints facing most medical institutions today impose limitations on the creation of training programs; nevertheless, several elements of the Children's Hospital program, particularly the in-service training and seminar, could be adapted to reduce their cost.

Clinical Training in Areas of Family Violence

Obviously, not all medical institutions have a Trauma X team or a Family Development Clinic to provide trainees with direct clinical experience in the area of child maltreatment. Nevertheless, most pediatric or family practice hospitals have services devoted to the treatment of injuries in children and are charged with the responsibility of recognizing and reporting child maltreatment. Such services can benefit from cooperation in postdoctoral training efforts designed to respond to the demands placed on medical institutions by laws relating to child abuse and neglect. Moreover, many such institutions have departments of psychiatry, and these departments can be a source of experienced personnel for supervising the clinical experience of trainees. In our own Family Violence Training Program at Children's Hospital, efforts to enlist the Department of Psychiatry to supervise fellows met with varying degrees of success. Appointing a psychologist from the Judge Baker Guidance Clinic as a program faculty member increased our ability to provide clinical supervision.

Whatever modifications must be made to accommodate the realities of other settings, five additional principles derived from our own experience with clinical training seem well worth considering. Our own efforts to establish a program guided by these principles have permeated this book. We hope that individuals in other settings will see the value of these principles and find ways to develop programs designed to follow them.

1. *Clinicians can benefit enormously from participation in an intellectual forum, from opportunities to leave the hurly-burly of the clinical environment and deal with each other in a personal way concerning issues of knowledge.* The clinical practice setting is often emotionally charged and fraught with conflicts across professional boundaries. Clinical data are highly complex, and dealing with these cases can be frustrating, even exhausting. The opportunity for a more intellectual perusal of issues related to clinical practice in an atmosphere that eases communication can provide a useful respite.

2. *Programs should find a way to provide clincians with research information that is directly relevant and helpful to their practice.* Even bright, sensitive, and caring clinicians can fall prey to such myths and stereotypes as the notion that if a home is neat and clean there is little likelihood of violence. During his year as a fellow, Richard Gelles repeatedly countered such clinical assumptions and beliefs with research data. His familiarity with research evidence finally persuaded clinicians that abuse is not just a parent-child phenomenon but can characterize a range of family interactions. With his input, clinicians learned to worry about how the mother got her black eye and not just about how the child became bruised. Clinicians often have had very inadequate training in the

area of family violence and can benefit greatly from exposure to knowledgeable reserchers in the field.

3. *Priority should be given to the perspectives and expertise of individuals in nursing and social services.* Professions with large proportions of women need to be empowered in medical environments. Often male-dominated professions have the most power and least perspective on problems such as interspousal violence. Such male-dominated professions tend to be symptom- and procedure-bound. By contrast, nurses and social workers tend to be more thoughtful, sensitive, and understanding; they attend to relationships. It is important to create ways for all professions, not just those traditionally female, to deal with subjective issues and to handle feelings and values.

4. *Links should be set up between the health-providing agencies and academic institutions.* Although adding such links may demand considerable time and effort on the part of individuals in both settings, the potential for payoff is also considerable in the form of professional enrichment and improved management of family violence. Hospitals can provide congenial settings in which academics can teach and learn from practitioners. Researchers and practitioners typically share a concern with promoting human welfare. Learning to speak each other's language and to cooperate in identifying and dealing with the human problems that pervade the medical setting is not impossible.

5. *It is important to promote positive relationships between health- and social service–providing agencies.* Seminars and interdisciplinary case conferences are useful means for bringing together people from different settings and for stimulating professional collaboration. Such opportunities for exchange and cooperation among professionals, whose responsibilities may differ greatly on a superficial and concrete level but converge when human welfare is considered on a more general level, can only enhance the effort to reduce the impact of family violence.

Appendixes

Appendix A
Child Abuse and Pediatric Social Illness:
An Epidemiological Analysis and Ecological Reformulation

Eli H. Newberger, M.D.
Robert L. Hampton, Ph.D.
Thomas J. Marx, Ed.D.
Kathleen M. White, Ed.D.

Children under four years of age hospitalized for child abuse, domestic accidents, failure to thrive, and ingestions were matched with controls admitted for comparably acute medical conditions. A structured parental interview yielded significant case-control differences. Discriminant analysis suggested interrelationships among the case groups, and cluster analysis identified three cohesive groups in terms of severity of symptoms. This reformulation provides a matrix for organizing data and an alternative to the present manifestational classification system.

The understanding of child abuse is limited by insufficient attention to issues of definition and etiology and by a particular

This work originally appeared in the *American Journal of Orthopsychiatry* 56, October 1986. Copyright © 1986 American Orthopsychiatric Association, Inc. Reproduced by permission.

focus on individual psychiatric disturbance.[19] The few existing controlled studies suggest that maltreatment has diverse concomitants in child development,[7] family stress,[18] parental and child conflicts,[3] and environmental difficulties.[10] Case-control studies, however, have been plagued with difficulties in achieving adequate matching, which lead in turn to confounding by social class and age and to forming causal inferences based on such commonly accepted risk factors as low birth weight, maternal depression, and the intergenerational transmission of violence.[12,17]

Advances in knowledge of child abuse suggest three areas in which past knowledge is challenged by newer findings and critical analyses. First, important associations may exist between violence toward children and violence between parents.[12,22] Second, the distinctive visibility, if not vulnerability, of poor, socially marginal, and minority children and families cannot be separated from a substantial bias which favors them for child abuse identification.[11-14,20,22] Third, the theoretical orientations of studies of child abuse define, select, and, to some extent, distort what we may understand as the nature, causes, and consequences of the problem: narrow and unitary conceptions of cause and effect may confine the available range of preventive and therapeutic interventions.[19]

More recent research appears to favor an ecological approach to child maltreatment, i.e., the progressive mutual adaptation of the individual and an environment conceptualized as a set of "nested" interactive systems.[2] Proponents of this ecological approach argue that we cannot ignore the influence of familial economic and demographic factors on the quality of life of children and their families.[1,5,8,9]

Ecological analysis focuses on the multiple levels of individual and family characteristics which interact with characteristics of the broader social context.[1,5,8,9] This approach to child abuse suggests, for example, that informal support networks can mediate the effects of economic stress, social isolation, and family structure by providing information, relief, and direct support. The existence of reciprocal helping relationships within a community appears to be associated with a lower prevalence of reported child abuse.[1,5,8,9] The framework argues for the collection and analysis of a rich array of data on child, family, and community.

The concept of pediatric social illness articulated previously[18] emphasizes the view that family environments and social conditions contribute importantly to the children's health and may form a common etiologic substrate for certain conditions. To understand more adequately the process by which a child might suffer inflicted trauma, accidental trauma, failure to thrive, or poisoning requires a capacity to organize the complex data that characterize a child's life setting.

The object of this investigation is to broaden the focus of inquiry with respect both to classification (from child abuse to pediatric social illness) and to the elements of risk (from personal pathologies to the family in its ecologic niche). Previous research on the pediatric social illnesses suggests that this conceptualization may be useful.[5,18]

Method

Sample

All children under four years of age hospitalized at Children's Hospital Medical Center, Boston, between July 1975 and April 1977 were eligible for selection as cases if they bore the diagnoses of child abuse, accident, ingestion, or nonorganic failure to thrive (FTT). Children hospitalized for comparably acute medical illnesses (such as pneumonia or meningitis) were eligible for selection as controls. Cases and controls were individually matched on three attributes: age, race, and socioeconomic status (determined by the Hollingshead two-factor social index).[15] The final sample consisted of 209 cases and 209 controls. Salient characteristics of the sample are presented in table A–1. A previous report compared the child developmental and family characteristics of the accident and child abuse victims in black families.[5]

Measures

The principal instrument was a standardized, precoded maternal interview lasting approximately one hour and conducted by specially

Table A–1
Sample Characteristics (N = 418)[1]

Variable	Percent	Variable	Percent
Child's Diagnosis		Age of Child	
Abuse	22.9	0 to 6 months	19.7
Failure to thrive	19.6	7 to 12 months	17.8
Accident	46.4	13 to 18 months	18.7
Ingestion	11.0	19 to 24 months	13.8
Sex of Child		25 months and older	30.1
Male	58.0	Child's Usual Health	
Female	42.0	Excellent	44.0
Race of Child		Good	39.0
White	69.0	Fair	13.0
Nonwhite	31.0	Poor	4.0
Family Receiving		Mother's Marital	
Public Assistance		Status	
Yes	45.0	Married	63.6
No	55.0	Single	19.3
		Separated, divorced	
		or widowed	16.9

[1]Each case was matched with a control of similar age, race, and SES. The sample contained a total of 209 cases and 209 controls.

trained interviewers at the hospital. (The interviewers were women with human service backgrounds, who were given supervision individually and in groups by two research psychologists. Although inter-interviewer reliability was not measured because of the constraints of the clinical setting, the systematic attention to interview technique and findings yielded an impression of a high order of reliability.) Questions focused on a wide range of variables including family structure, housing, employment, finances, support, mobility, psychological stresses, child rearing, and the parents' own childhoods. Data on the child included a Vineland Social Maturity Index derived from a maternal report. Carey's adaptation of the Thomas, Chess, and Birch infant scales was employed to assess the mother's perceptions of her child's temperament.[4,23] From the medical records, physical characteristics were obtained, i.e., height, weight, hematocrit, head circumference, and duration of hospitalization.

Data Analysis

First, we examined each of the independent variables separately in relation to each group of pediatric social illness cases and their matched controls in order to define the associations and their directions. We accomplished this step with a series of cross-tabulations and used *t*-tests and chi-square tests respectively to assess statistical significance for continuous and categorical variables (see table A–2). Next, we used discriminant analysis to determine from all the variables which set of variables—together and relative to others—provided the best means of discriminating cases from controls.

Finally, we employed hierarchical cluster analysis to search for homogeneous groups, irrespective of diagnosis, in a random half-sample of the entire population, and we replicated this analysis on the other half-sample.

Discriminant Function Analyses

The most important results of the four multiple discriminant function (MDF) equations we constructed can be seen in table A–3, which summarizes the variables that emerged as the most powerful discriminators between each case category and its controls, and lists the variables considered for entry by the MDF program. Characteristics of the children served in all instances to differentiate between cases and controls. Child characteristics, aspects of the parent-child relationship, past stresses, and life-context variables emerged as significant variables in some but not all of the discriminant function equations.

Although we found evidence that all categories of pediatric social illness are characterized by some isolation of case families from their kin and communities, this isolation was most pervasive in the families that bear the diagnosis of abuse. Of the 18 variables that entered the abuse discriminant function equation at a significance level of 0.05 or more, seven reflected directly the mother's current social isolation. An eighth variable, recent death of a family member, may contribute to isolation as well as to general stress.

Table A–2
Attributes of Cases and Matched Controls

Variable	Cases (N = 48)	Controls (N = 48)	Total
Child Abuse			
Mother has Telephone			
Yes	59.4%	40.6%	35.6%
No	37.9	62.1	64.4
$\chi^2 = 3.8$; $df = 1$; $p \leq .05$			
Child Easy or Difficult			
Very difficult	64.0	36.0	28.1
Not very difficult	39.1	60.9	71.9
$\chi^2 = 4.5$; $df = 1$; $p \leq .03$			
Times/Week Spanks Child			
Zero	53.7	46.3	61.4
One to three	47.1	52.9	19.3
Four or more	17.7	82.4	19.3
$\chi^2 = 6.8$; $df = 2$; $p \leq .03$			
Mother's Description of Childhood			
Unhappy	85.7	14.3	15.7
Slightly unhappy	44.0	56.0	28.1
Slightly happy	45.0	55.0	22.5
Very happy	30.0	70.0	33.7
$\chi^2 = 12.0$; $df = 3$; $p \leq .007$			
Maternal Grandmother's Discipline Felt			
Severe	75.0	25.0	29.3
Appropriate	33.0	66.7	58.5
Lenient	40.0	60.0	12.2
$\chi^2 = 11.4$; $df = 2$; $p \leq .003$			
Mother Rural to Urban Shift			
Yes	52.8	47.2	80.0
No	16.7	83.3	20.0
$\chi^2 = 7.6$; $df = 1$; $p \leq .006$			
Father Rural to Urban Shift			
Yes	30.2	69.8	47.8
No	59.6	40.4	52.2
$\chi^2 = 7.8$; $df = 1$; $p \leq .005$			
Child Below Age Self-help, Dressing			
Yes	80.0	20.0	11.6
No	39.5	60.5	88.4
$\chi^2 = 5.9$; $df = 1$; $p \leq .02$			
Child Below Age of Communication			
Behind	63.6	36.4	25.6
Not behind	37.5	62.5	74.4
$\chi^2 = 4.5$; $df = 1$; $p \leq .03$			

Table A–2 continued

Variable	Cases (N = 48)	Controls (N = 48)	Total
Times/Week Mother Sees Relatives			
Once	65.5%	36.0%	27.8%
Twice	52.0	48.0	27.6
Three times or more	25.0	75.0	40.2
$\chi^2 = 11.2$; $df = 2$; $p \leq .03$			
Mother Sees Relatives Enough			
Yes	40.3	59.7	87.5
No	81.8	18.2	12.5
$\chi^2 = 6.7$; $df = 1$; $p \leq .01$			
Failure to Thrive	(N – 41)	(N – 41)	
Mother Owns Car			
Yes	41.7%	58.3%	55.2%
No	66.7	33.3	44.8
$\chi^2 = 5.4$; $df = 1$; $p \leq .02$			
Child's Usual Health			
Poor to fair	79.0	21.5	22.6
Good	65.8	34.2	45.2
Excellent	22.2	77.8	32.1
$\chi^2 = 17.9$; $df = 2$; $p \leq .0001$			
Times/Month Mother Has Headaches			
None	41.5	58.5	47.7
One to seven	70.6	29.4	39.5
More than seven	45.5	54.6	12.8
$\chi^2 = 6.7$; $df = 2$; $p \leq .04$			
Mother's Emotional Support			
Enough	59.4	40.6	82.1
Sometimes enough	27.3	72.7	13.1
Not enough	0.0	100.0	3.6
None	100.0	0.0	1.2
$\chi^2 = 8.3$; $df = 3$; $p \leq .04$			
Child Below Age Locomotion			
Yes	92.3	7.7	15.3
No	48.6	51.4	84.7
$\chi^2 = 8.5$; $df = 1$; $p \leq .03$			
Number of Categories Behind Age Group			
Zero	50.0	50.0	44.7
One	29.2	70.8	28.2
Two	92.9	7.1	16.5
Three or more	100.0	0.0	10.6
$\chi^2 = 20.1$; $df = 4$; $p \leq .03$			

Table A–2 continued

Variable	Cases (N = 48)	Controls (N = 48)	Total
Vineland Social Quotient			
Low	80.0%	20.0%	29.8%
High	45.8	54.2	70.2
$\chi^2 = 6.9$; $df = 2$; $p \leq .03$			

	Cases (N = 97)	Controls (N = 97)	Total
Accident			
Times/Week Mother Sees Relatives			
No relatives	30.0%	70.0%	15.9%
Rarely	48.3	51.7	30.7
Sometimes	59.7	40.4	30.2
Often	68.8	31.3	8.5
Very often	42.9	57.1	14.8
$\chi^2 = 9.8$; $df = 4$; $p \leq .04$			
Child's Usual Health			
Poor to fair	20.8	79.2	12.6
Good	45.3	54.7	39.3
Excellent	60.9	39.1	48.2
$\chi^2 = 14.6$; $df = 3$; $p \leq .002$			
Religion Specified			
Yes	45.2	54.8	81.4
No	69.4	30.6	18.6
$\chi^2 = 6.9$; $df = 1$; $p \leq .01$			

	Cases (N = 23)	Controls (N = 23)	Total
Ingestion			
Below Age Communication			
Behind	100.0%	0.0%	11.1%
Not behind	42.5	57.5	88.9
$\chi^2 = 5.9$; $df = 1$; $p \leq .02$			
Below Age Any Category			
Behind	70.6	29.4	37.0
Not behind	37.9	62.1	63.0
$\chi^2 = 4.6$; $df = 1$; $p \leq .03$			
Extended Family			
No	56.4	43.6	84.8
Yes	14.3	85.7	15.2
$\chi^2 = 4.2$; $df = 1$; $p \leq .04$			

Note: Full contingency tables omitted because of space limitations. Percentages may not add to 100 because of rounding.

Stresses differed between mothers of abused children and their controls. The former may have seen their relatives less often, felt that no one was interested in their problems, have suffered a recent death in the family, coped alone with child care, and disagreed with their husbands concerning discipline and child rearing. They could count on few relatives to help and had fewer kin in their communities. More than the mothers in the other case categories, they appeared to see themselves as unconnected to others.

Past stresses entered the discriminant function equations at significant levels only for ingestion and abuse cases. Mothers of abuse victims reported unhappy childhoods.

Aspects of the parent-child relationship entered discriminant function equations at significant levels for both accident and abuse victims. Paradoxically, the mothers of abuse victims reported spanking their children less than mothers in other case categories. Although this report may be untruthful, betrayed by the diagnosis, and forced by the hospital context in which the interview was conducted, lack of truthfulness is not the only hypothesis to arise from this finding. Previous study of the interaction between abuse victims and their parents, for example, disclose interaction patterns that included a high degree of both permissiveness and punitiveness.[24] Indeed, the frequency of hitting might have been less, but the child's provocations might have been met with more severe violence. In the Sears, Maccoby, and Levin study of child-rearing patterns, this parenting style was associated with the most frequent expression of serious aggression in children's observed play.[21]

We also noted significant case-control distinctions between the accident victims' mothers' reports of striking the child on vulnerable body parts and the age at which a child could reasonably be expected to be toilet trained. These reports, more commonly associated with clinical and investigative work on abused children, suggest the possibility that a parent's capacity to protect a child from anger may be connected to the capacity to protect the child from environmental hazards. Preschool children's own propensities for accidents may be increased by the child's inability to internalize self-protection, even as the child is not protected by the parent; the possibly exaggerated expectations of the child may indicate a diagnostic overlap with child abuse in more than a few cases.

Mothers of both accident and abuse victims came more frequently from urban areas and they specified their religions less

Table A–3

Discriminant Function Analysis: Variables Discriminating between Each Case Category and Its Controls

Accident   (N = 194)
Few medical visits in last year***
Recent moves***
Healthy
Religion specified less often**
Child spanked more often than on hands
    and bottom*
Mother's family residence in urban area**
Mother estimates young age for toilet training*
Advocacy needs higher*
Relatives seen less often
Less access to shopping and recreation
Fewer social agencies
Mother less likely to be born in U.S.
    Wilkes Lambda: .739
    Canonical R: .510

Failure to Thrive   (N = 82)
Unhealthy***
Reactive to visual and auditory changes**
Mother sees relatives less often per week*
Mothers gets away by self less often*
Mother watches TV more*
Mother has fewer adult relatives in Boston
Advocacy needs higher
Mother less likely to have own car

Ingestion   (N = 46)
Low Vineland Social Maturity score**
Healthy*
Extended family unavailable*
Mother gets away by self less often
As a child, mother was more often spanked
    with objects
Advocacy needs higher
    Wilkes Lambda: .461
    Canonical R: .733

Abuse   (N = 96)
Mother sees relatives less per week***
Mother's childhood unhappy***
Mother reports spanking child less**
Mother feels no one interested in problems*
Child easy or difficult*
Fewer months since mother had last job
Religion specified less often
Recent death in family*
More social agencies*
Mother's family residence in urban area*
Mother doesn't see relatives enough**
Mother less likely to have own car
Mother and father disagree on discipline**
Little help with child care*

Low Vineland Social Maturity score**	
Mother spanked more often than on hands and bottom**	
Mother has fewer relatives in Boston*	
Mother and father disagree on childrearing	
Wilkes Lambda:	.141
Canonical R:	.926
When mother and father disagree, more likely to hit and throw objects	
Wilkes Lambda:	.423
Canonical R:	.832

*p<.05 **p<.01 ***p<.001.

Note: Variables listed in order of their inclusion.

Variables Entered into the Multiple Discriminant Function Program: Times week mother sees relatives (*Abuse, Accidents*); Mother describes childhood as happy (*Abuse*); Times week mother spanks child (*Abuse, FTT*); Mother feels no one interested in her problems (*Abuse, Accidents*); Child easy or difficult (*Abuse, Accidents*); Months since mother's last ob (*Abuse, Accidents*); Religion specified (*Abuse, Accidents*); Parent recent death stressful (*Abuse, FTT, Accidents*); Times month mother has headaches (*Abuse*); Mother's family intact (*Abuse*); Number of social agencies (*Abuse, Accidents*); Mother happy with pregnancy (*Abuse*); Mother's family residence urban area (*Abuse, Accidents*); Mother born in U.S. (*Abuse, Accidents*); Mother and father disagree violently (*Abuse, FTT, Accidents*); Mother sees relatives enough (*Abuse, Ingestions*); Parents consider neighborhood safe (*Abuse*); Mother owns car (*Abuse*); Mother's number of friends in neighborhood (*Abuse*); Child reacts to new foods (*Abuse*); Mother and father disagree on discipline (*Abuse, FTT, Accidents*); Marital status (*Abuse*); Mother's number of relatives in city (*Abuse, Accidents*); Age of mother (*Abuse, Accidents*); Child premature (*Abuse*); Mother's parents agree on childrearing (*Abuse*); Mother physically punished in childhood (*Abuse, Ingestions*); Times child at MD last year (*Accidents*); Child's usual health (*FTT, Accidents, Ingestions*); Child's reactivity to auditory and visual stimuli (*Abuse, FTT*); Child's tempo of play (*FTT*); Total number of children in family (*FTT*); Male present (*FTT*); Social isolation (*FTT, Ingestions*); Mother's education (*FTT, Accidents*); Family stress (*FTT*); Maternal use of drugs and alcohol (*FTT*); Child's sleep pattern (*FTT*); Difficult child to feed (*FTT*); Unhappy maternal childhood (*Abuse, FTT*); Times per week child is spanked (*FTT, Ingestions*); Number of moves within last year (*FTT, Accidents*); Planned vs. unplanned pregnancy (*FTT*); Mother views current relationship as supportive (*FTT*); Parents agree on childrearing practices (*FTT*); Mother's usual health (*FTT*); Mother sees herself as happy (*FTT*); Mother has telephone (*Abuse, Ingestions*); Total family advocacy needs (*Ingestions, Accidents*); Mother just can't get going (*Accidents*); Private pediatrician (*Accidents*); Childrearing problems (*Accidents*); Mother spanked Mother's ease to shopping and recreation (*Accidents*); Extended family available (*Abuse, FTT, Ingestions, Accidents*); Child's locomotion skills (*FTT*).

often. In additon, the mothers of abuse victims were in contact substantially more with social agencies than their controls or the mothers of the accident victims.

The correct classification yielded by the multiple discriminant analyses are presented in table A–4. Application of the abuse equation to the abuse sample and its controls resulted in correct classification of 92% of the abuse cases and 90% of their controls. Application of the failure-to-thrive equation to the failure-to-thrive cases and their controls resulted in correct classification of 76% of the FTT cases and 88% of their controls. The ingestion equation yielded correct classification of 87% of the ingestion cases and 87% of their controls, and the accident equation yielded correct classification of 76% of the accident cases and 71% of their controls.

As a result of this study, in which we examined how pediatric social illness categories differed and overlapped, we examined whether an alternative to the traditional pediatric classification might provide a more informative grouping of cases and controls.

Table A–4
Correct and Incorrect Classification of Cases
from Discriminant Function Analysis

	Predicted Group	
Actual Group	*Cases*	*Controls*
Accident		
Cases $(N=97)$	76%	24%
Controls $(N=97)$	29	71
Ingestion		
Cases $(N=23)$	87	13
Controls $(N=23)$	13	87
Failure to Thrive		
Cases $(N=41)$	76	24
Controls $(N=41)$	12	88
Abuse		
Cases $(N=48)$	92	8
Controls $(N=48)$	10	90

Hierarchical Cluster Analysis

Discriminant analyses allowed us to differentiate between groups based on our existing diagnostic categories. In contrast, cluster analysis generated new categorical schemes by partitioning a set of cases into homogeneous subgroups. Hierarchical cluster analysis permitted us to explore the extent to which natural clusters may exist within our data set.

We performed a cluster analysis on a random half-sample of cases in our study. The 63 variables upon which the half-sample was clustered made up the set that best discriminated cases from controls within each of the pediatric social illness categories as well as the set of variables that discriminated families bearing the abuse diagnosis from families bearing the accident diagnosis. Before analysis could take place, each variable was transformed into standard scores (Z-Scores).

The initial cluster analysis produced six cohesive clusters, containing 202 of the 209 families. The remaining families could not be placed in any specific cluster. We used a similar procedure on the second half-sample; 199 of 209 families fell into one of six clusters. Even though six clusters were formed for each subsample, the primary test for validity was whether we discovered similar clusters across subsamples.

We designed a threefold procedure to determine whether the same clusters appeared across both subsets. First, to be paired, two clusters had to distribute identically, within sampling fluctuation, over the five diagnostic outcomes. Second, a comparison of mean values for two clusters across the 63 variables had to yield few statistical differences. Third, the two clusters had to be relatively similar in size.

Two clusters from the original and reserve half-samples paired handsomely. Their distributions on diagnoses were very close; means did not significantly differ on 59 of the 63 cluster variables, and they were of similar sizes (90 and 92). This group of 182, which turned out to be at lowest risk for abuse or failure to thrive, we called the ecologic advantage group.

The clusters that formed our group at highest risk for abuse or failure to thrive also paired well, with one exception. They too were distributed very similarly over the diagnoses, but with very low counts for most diagnoses, and their means did not differ on 56 out of the 63 cluster variables. Sample sizes, however, were statistically discrepant. The cluster from the original sample included eight families, whereas the cluster from the reserve sample included 18. Despite the discrepancy in subcluster size, this group became our ecologic crisis group.

A third subgroup was formed by combining one group from our original and two from the reserve sample. This cluster was somewhat less homogeneous than the others, though both samples were similar with respect to their distributions across categories of pediatric social illness. These 112 cases constituted our ecologic adversity cluster.

Figure A–1 shows histograms of diagnoses for each of the three risk groups. Note the distribution of abuse and failure to thrive among the three groups. While 37% of families in the ecologic crisis cluster were diagnosed as abusive, only 7% of families in the adversity and advantage clusters were so diagnosed. Thus, abuse among the families in ecologic crisis was five times as prevalent as among the other two groups combined. While 23% of children in the crisis cluster were diagnosed as failure to thrive, 13% of families in the other two groups were so diagnosed. Thus, failure to thrive among families in ecologic crisis was about 1.5 times as prevalent as among the ecologic adversity and advantage groups.

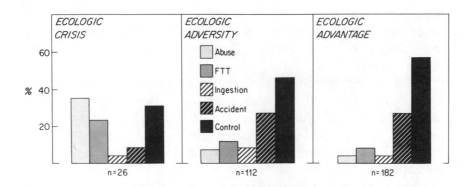

Figure A–1. *Cluster Composition*

The picture is reversed for accidents and acute medical conditions. Only 8% of children in the crisis group were classified as accidents, whereas 37% of the children in the adversity and advantage groups were identified as accidents, about 4.5 times as many as in the crisis cluster. Acute medical conditions were 2.3 times as prevalent in the adversity and advantage groups as in the crisis group.

Group Profiles Analyses

For each of the 63 variables that defined interfamilial distance and (taken together) formed the three clusters, we executed a one-way analysis of variance (ANOVA) followed by a Duncan Multiple Range Test. The *F*-test and R-square from the ANOVA, shown on table A–5, demonstrated how well each variable differentiated the three groups. The Duncan Test answered a more refined question: for the variable under study and for each of the three possible pairings of two groups, did the two groups differ at or below the 0.05 level of significance?[6,16]

For any set of three tests of a variable based on three pairings, the probability of not erroneously declaring a random difference significant is 0.95. Across the entire set of 189 Duncan tests, however, this probability drops to 0.04. Therefore, it is reasonably certain that at least one of our findings is wrong. But the probability that no more than seven significant results are false is 0.99. On the basis of these error rates, we may say that a few of the differences set forth below are likely to be spurious, but the great majority of them are not.

High-Risk Family Profile

Family Wealth

Whether family wealth is measured by income or by welfare dependency, families in the ecologic crisis cluster were poor. Even though families in the other clusters were by no means affluent, their mean family incomes were more than twice the mean family

Table A-5
Analysis of Variance for Cluster Variables

Variable	F-Value	R^2
Per capita income	9.4***	.055
Welfare	23.8***	1.30
Mother has own car	30.7***	.162
Mother describes childhood as happy	12.8***	.074
Maternal grandmother ever hit elsewhere than bottom or hand	38.8***	.196
Maternal grandmother's discipline appropriate	39.2***	.198
Maternal grandparents agreed on childrearing	12.8***	.074
Mother was hit into adolescence	31.9***	.167
Mother's education	19.5***	.109
Mother's occupation	33.0***	.172
Mother's health problems	40.5***	.203
Mother just can't get going	11.6***	.068
Hours mother watches TV	21.7***	.120
Mother feels no one interested in problems	3.7*	.022
Mother describes living situation as happy	7.3***	.044
Recent death stressful	7.1**	.042
Marital status	40.2***	.202
Male present	19.3***	.108
Mother's years single	7.4**	.044
Mother's number of relatives can count on	34.9***	.180
Mother's ease to bus	3.9*	.023
Child's health	11.4***	.067
Vineland social quotient	22.7***	.125
Hematocrit	3.9*	.024
Below age of self-help in general	10.3***	.060
Below age of communication	4.5*	.027
Below age of socialization	12.7***	.074

*p<.05; **p<.01; ***p<.001.

income of the crisis cluster. Data with respect to welfare dependency reinforced this income picture. Seven of eight families in the crisis cluster received public assistance, but only one out of three in the advantaged families and one out of six families in the adversity cluster received welfare.

Mother's Childhood

The parents of mothers in families in ecologic crisis often disagreed about child rearing, according to the mother. These mothers remembered being disciplined more severely than mothers in the other groups. They were more often hit with objects, and on parts of the body other than hands or buttocks. In many cases physical discipline continued into adolescence. When asked to summarize their childhoods, mothers in the crisis group gave a neutral assessment, in contrast to other mothers who felt that they were "somewhat happy" as children.

Mother's Attainments

The more skilled the mother's occupation, the less risk there appeared to be that her child would be diagnosed as abused or failing to thrive. In order from highest to lowest risk groups, the mothers' occupations were: unskilled or semiskilled labor, skilled labor, and clerical work. This pattern was repeated for education. Among families in crisis, mothers had rarely finished high school. More education was associated significantly with a more favored ecologic state.

Mother's State

Mothers in the crisis cluster reported minor to moderate health problems while other mothers voiced few health complaints. In addition to health problems, many high-risk mothers sometimes had difficulty in getting started in the morning, as suggested in their reports of watching an average of $7^1/_2$ hours of television per day. Mothers in the other adversity and advantage clusters watched $3^1/_2$ and 3 hours of television per day respectively.

Mothers in the crisis cluster appeared to be more beset by physical and psychological problems. They were also more likely to feel, at least some of the time, that no one cared what happened to them. In addition, only slightly more than half described themselves as happy, while over 80% of mothers in the lower-risk groups felt they were happy.

Mother's Relationships

In almost all families in crisis, the mothers were single, separated, or divorced. This absence of a partner diminished as advantage increased; the married state differentiated significantly among the groups. In homes of crisis, there was either no man or a man who did not always live there. More often than not, advantaged mothers were living with a man to whom, most frequently, they were married.

The data also suggest that the more kin one has available, the greater the ecologic advantage.

Mothers in the crisis cluster claimed that they spanked no more than mothers in the other two groups. These mothers, however, found their children more difficult to manage than lower-risk mothers.

Child's State

The evidence of the child's state was taken from the mother's impression after admission of the child to the hospital as a patient. Her interview response might have been influenced by her reactions to doctors, nurses, or social workers who had conferred with her about the child.

Mothers in the crisis group appraised their child's usual health as less favorable than mothers in the other groups. The Vineland Social Maturity Score was also calculated from information given by the mother. The more advantaged children enjoyed higher scores.

The hematocrits (percentage of red blood cells in centrifugal whole blood) of children in the crisis cluster were slightly lower than the hematocrits of children in the other two groups, but they were not so low that these children, as a group, could be called anemic. Children in the three groups reacted similarly to visual and auditory changes, and they were similarly distractable during fussy periods.

Father's Background

Though most fathers of families in ecologic crisis were raised in rural locations, most fathers in the two other groups were raised in urban locations. In addition, slightly higher rates of broken marriage were found between parents of fathers in families in crisis.

Discussion

Children admitted to a pediatric hospital with diagnoses of abuse, accidents, ingestions, and nonorganic failure to thrive differed from children with comparably acute medical conditions not only on the basis of presenting symptomatology but also on the basis of a variety of ecological characteristics. Regardless of the particular assigned diagnosis, families of children with a social illness appeared on the whole to be experiencing more stresses in their lives than the families of children with nonfatal acute medical conditions.

Cluster analysis confirmed our notion that abusing families were not characterized by a distinct constellation of variables that set them apart totally from families of children with other diagnoses. Indeed, cases of abuse, like cases of nonorganic failure to thrive, appear in all three of the clusters—ecologic advantage, ecologic adversity, and ecologic crisis—that emerged, although in very different proportions. Information in depth on the children's family circumstances is essential to define the nature and extent of an individual child's vulnerability and risk.

Our profile of high-risk families in certain vital areas of their lives—family wealth, mother's childhood, mother's attainments, mother's state, mother's relationships, child's state, and father's background—revealed that, in nearly every domain, the crisis cluster appears to suffer. Whether or not abuse or failure to thrive had occurred in these families, they usually had woefully inadequate financial means and major problems in intimate relationships. The mother's entire life may have been impoverished and punctuated by violence and abandonment.

The three empirically derived clusters identified in this study provide a matrix for organizing data from families whose children suffer pediatric social illnesses. They do not imply judgment of a parent's adequacy, but rather they focus on specific aspects of family functioning in the life setting. We believe practice will improve when, with compassion and respect, clinicians can systematically identify and address the strengths and weaknesses of parents, children, and nurturing environments.

References

1. Belsky, J. 1980. Child maltreatment: an ecological integration. Amer. Psychol. 35:320–335.
2. Bronfenbrenner, U. 1979. The Ecology of Human Development. Harvard University Press, Cambridge.

3. Burgess, R.; and Conger, R. 1978. Family interaction in abusive, neglectful, and normal families. Child Devlpm. 49:163–173.
4. Carey, W. 1970. A simplified method for measuring infant temperament. J. Pediat. 188–194.
5. Daniel, J., Hampton, R., and Newberger, E. 1983. Child abuse and childhood accidents in black families: a controlled comparative study. Amer. J. Orthopsychiat. 53:645–653.
6. Duncan, D. 1975. T-tests and intervals for comparison suggested by the data. Biometrics 31:339–359.
7. Friedrich, W., and Einbender, A. 1983. The abused child: a psychological review. J. Clin. Child Psychol. 12:244–256.
8. Garbarino, J. 1977. The human ecology of child maltreatment: a conceptual model for research, J. Marr. Fam. 39:721–736.
9. Garbarino, J. 1982. Children and Families in the Social Environment. Aldine, New York.
10. Garbarino, J., and Crouter, A. 1978. Defining the community context for parent-child relations: the correlates of child maltreatment. Child Devlpm. 49:604–616.
11. Gelles, R. 1979. Community agencies and child abuse: labeling and gatekeeping. In Family Violence, R. Gelles, ed. Sage Publications, Beverly Hills, Calif.
12. Gelles, R. 1980. Violence in the family: a review of research in the seventies. J. Marr. Fam. 42:875–885.
13. Gelles, R. 1982. Child abuse and family violence: implications for medical professionals. In Child Abuse, E. Newberger, ed. Little, Brown, Boston.
14. Hampton, R., and Newberger, E. 1985. Child abuse incidents and reporting by hospitals: significance of severity, class and race. Amer. J. Pub. Hlth 75:56–60.
15. Hollingshead, A., and Redlich, F. 1958. Social Class and Mental Illness. John Wiley, New York.
16. Miller, R. 1981. Simultaneous Statistical Inference. Springer Verlag, New York.
17. Newberger, E., and Daniel, J. 1976. Knowledge and epidemiology of child abuse: a critical review of concepts. Pediat. Ann. 5:140–144.
18. Newberger, E., et al. 1977. Pediatric social illness: toward an etiologic classification. Pediatrics 60:178–185.
19. Newberger, E., Newberger, C., and Hampton, R. 1983. Child abuse: the current theory base and future research needs. J. Amer. Acad. Child Psychiat. 22:262–268.
20. O'Toole, R., Turbett, P., and Nalepka, C. 1983. Theories, professional knowledge and diagnosis of child abuse. In The Dark Side of Families: Current Family Violence Research, D. Finkelhor, et al., eds. Sage Publications, Beverly Hills, Calif.
21. Sears, R., Maccoby, E., and Levin, H. 1957. Patterns of Child Rearing. Row and Peterson, Evanston, Ill.

22. Straus, M., Gelles, R., and Steinmetz, S. 1980. Behind Closed Doors: Violence in the American Family. Doubleday, New York.
23. Thomas, A., Chess, S., and Birch, H. 1978. Temperament and Behavior Disorders in Children. New York University Press, New York.
24. Wasserman, G., Green, A., and Allen, R. 1983. Going beyond abuse: maladaptive patterns of interaction in abusing mother-infant pairs. J. Amer. Acad. Child Psychiat. 22:245–252.

Appendix B
Consensus and Difference among Hospital Professionals in Evaluating Child Maltreatment

Jane C. Snyder
Eli H. Newberger

The decision-making process in suspected cases of child maltreatment involves reaching interprofessional consensus. Interprofessional consensus in seriousness ratings of maltreatment incidents for the welfare of the child was examined by surveying 39 case vignette ratings by 295 pediatric hospital professionals from five occupations. The survey instrument was derived from research by Giovannoni and Becerra (1979). An exploratory factor analysis yielded five categories of maltreatment: physical abuse, sexual abuse, general failures in care, minor neglect/discipline, and life-style/values. A sixth category, parental sexual preference, was rated not very serious and did not appear to belong in the maltreatment domain. Nurses and social workers rated incidents as most serious, differing significantly from psychiatrists and, often, from physicians and psychologists. Professions agreed on rank ordering of categories by seriousness. Variables such as sex, parenthood status, years of experience, and medical specialty showed some relationship to ratings within some professional groups.

This work originally appeared in *Violence and Victims 1*, No. 2, 1986, © Copyright 1986 by Springer Publishing Co., Inc., New York. Used by permission.

Medical and mental health professionals and educators are mandated by law to identify and report cases of suspected child maltreatment. Identifying such cases is not an easy task. A number of clinicians have written on the emotional and situational concomitants of identification and reporting (e.g., Elmer, 1960; Helfer, 1975; Hill, 1975; Rosenfeld & Newberger, 1977; Rosenzweig, 1982). Definitions of child abuse in state reporting statutes list general areas of concern such as physical abuse, physical neglect, sexual abuse, emotional abuse, and educational and medical neglect. The vague nature of these definitions contributes to difficulty in case identification.

Defining specific constituents of abuse or neglect is left to the professional. Filing a report of suspected maltreatment initiates an investigation by the state's protective services division, resulting in further definition; the case is either "substantiated" or closed. State agency guidelines regarding which cases will be substantiated are as likely to change with budget considerations as with attention to conditions adversely affecting children (Newberger et al., 1975).

Many have argued that applying the label of child abuse or neglect implies a judgment about social deviance and brings to bear both personal and societal values regarding parenting (e.g., Gelles, 1973; Giovannoni & Becerra, 1979; Nagi, 1977). Implicit in the process of defining child abuse are judgments about circumstances harmful to children, minimal requirements for adequate child development, and aspects of a child or person that are most important for society to protect. Such judgments may be affected by a number of subjective variables, including: personal experience as a child and parent (Kaufman, 1983), social group affiliation and accompanying norms for appropriate child care (Daniel, 1985; Korbin, 1977), and personal values (Rosenzweig, 1985). It is also likely that the professional training one has received will affect the standard used in defining maltreatment, as different occupational groups have different roles in working with children and families, and concern themselves with different aspects of child development.

Several research studies have investigated differences among professional groups in assigning the label of child abuse to case vignettes (Gelles, 1975; Nalepka, O'Toole & Turbett, 1981; Turbett

& O'Toole, 1980). Differences among professionals in these studies were most apparent on vignettes which presented ambiguous intentionality of action on the part of the caretaker, and in cases where effects on the child were not obvious. High agreement occurred on "the outrageous cases," e.g., cigarette burns (Gelles, 1975). However, these studies and others (e.g., Hampton & Newberger, 1985; Katz et al., 1986) have documented that factors such as race and social class are as important in determining which cases will be labeled as child maltreatment and in affecting the disposition of those cases, as is the nature of the injury or incident, particularly given ambiguous circumstances.

Many pediatric hospitals employ interdisciplinary teams to facilitate the decision-making process in suspected cases and to guard against the subjective bias of any one individual or professional viewpoint. If a formal team does not exist, an informal case management conference may be held. The difficulties in arriving at consensus, documented in research studies, have also been observed in clinical practice (e.g., Bourne & Newberger, 1980), where most cases are, in fact, ambiguous.[1] The greater the extent of disagreement among team members, the more difficult it becomes to devise an adequate case plan.

In this study, the degree of consensus among occupational groups involved in clinical decision making in suspected cases of child abuse was investigated in a pediatric hospital setting. The survey instrument was adapted from methodology used in a study of the child abuse definition process (Giovannoni & Becerra, 1979), in which participants were asked to assess seriousness for the welfare of the child in 78 case vignettes.

Giovannoni and Becerra studied five professional groups: social workers, police, pediatricians, lawyers, and a lay sample. Significant disagreement among professional groups occurred on all but nine vignettes. All groups tended to agree in *relative* ranking of categories of maltreatment by seriousness—rating physical abuse, sexual abuse, and the fostering of delinquency as most serious. "Educational neglect and failure to provide" preceded "parental sexual mores," which were viewed as least serious. Inadequate supervision and emotional maltreatment were rated between the two extremes.

Giovannoni and Becerra used two forms, with one set of vignettes adding consequences for the child. This addition significantly increased the ratings of seriousness for over half the vignettes, decreased ratings for nine, and made no difference in 26 cases. Relative ranking according to seriousness remained the same with and without consequences, however. Medical neglect was the category in which professionals were most affected by the addition of consequences. In this category, seriousness ratings decreased for pediatricians and increased for the other groups.

Since the general findings were the same with and without consequences, and since knowledge of consequences is part of the information used in clinical decision making in hospital settings, vignettes used in the present study included this dimension.

Method

Subjects

Members of five professional groups at an urban pediatric teaching hospital and an affiliated mental health clinic participated in the study: physicians (nonpsychiatrists), nurses, social workers, psychologists, and psychiatrists. Physicians, psychiatrists, and psychologists were surveyed at the start of in-service teaching sessions on child abuse or related topics at the hospital or affiliated clinic. Nurses and social workers were surveyed in two ways: 64% ($N = 53$) of the social workers and 36% ($N = 31$) of the nurses were contacted at the beginning of in-service teaching sessions. In order to obtain more participants from these groups, the questionnaire was mailed to all hospital social workers and social work students and to nursing staff on hospital divisions frequently involved with child abuse cases. A 60% response rate ($N = 30$) was obtained from social work staff, and 40% ($N = 56$) from nursing staff. (The social work sample included 14 protective social workers attending a hospital teaching conference. Their responses were analyzed separately from the rest of the social work group but did not differ significantly and were combined into the total sample.)

Of the 306 returned questionnaires, 295 met the study criteria, i.e., were complete, and came from professionals within the five disciplines. Tables B–1 and B–2 summarize subject characteristics for each professional group, including sex, age, parenthood status, years of experience posttraining, and prior involvement with cases of abuse or neglect.

Instrument

A questionnaire was constructed utilizing 39 of the 78 case vignettes from the Giovannoni and Becerra study (1979). Vignettes were chosen that maximally discriminated among professional groups within each of the 13 categories defined a priori by Giovannoni and Becerra. Four introductory vignettes were included, representing the range of seriousness for situations presented. Introductory vignettes included instances of verbal abuse, medical neglect, physical abuse, and physical and sexual abuse. All vignettes were two sentences in length and included a description of the act and of the consequences for the child.

Sample vignettes:

1. The parents make their child steal small items from a supermarket. The child was caught stealing.
2. The parents and child have engaged in sexual intercourse. The child has gonorrhea.
3. The parents somtimes leave their child alone all night. The child is afraid of intruders.

Table B–1
*Percentage of Males and Females in
Each Professional Group*

Profession	(N)	Males (%)	Females (%)
Nurses	87	1	99
Social workers	83	17	83
Psychologists	32	25	75
Physicians	78	71	29
Psychiatrists	15	80	20
Total sample	295	31	69

Table B–2
Personal Characteristics by Profession

Characteristic	Total Sample	Nurses	Social Workers	Psychologists	Physicians	Psychiatrists
			Profession			
Mean age (yr)	33	34	32	32	31	42
% who are parents	32	31	31	33	23	73
% with involvement in case	48	75	16	33	45	73
Mean years of experi- ence posttraining	6.5	7.8	5.5	4.0	a	9.9
N	295	87	83	32	78	15

[a]Given the large number of physicians in training, the mean is not informative. See note 2.

Subjects were instructed to assume that the child was 7 years old and to rate the seriousness of the situation for the child's welfare on a 9-point scale (9 = very serious, 1 = not very serious).

Data Analysis

The data analysis proceeded in three steps. First, the data were factor analyzed to determine categories of maltreatment. Second, an analysis of professional differences in seriousness ratings on individual items and factors was performed using one-way analyses of variance. Third, the relationship of other subject variables to seriousness ratings was analyzed.

Results

Factor Analysis

A factor structure was predicted based on the Giovannoni and Beccrra 9-factor structure. The predicted structure was not confirmed by confirmatory factor analysis of these data. An exploratory factor analysis with Varimax rotation was then performed. Six factors emerged from this analysis, explaining 70% of the variance. Table B–3 lists the items and factor loadings. The factors, in order of variance accounted for, were: general failures in care, parental sexual preference, sexual abuse, physical abuse, minor neglect and discipline, and life-style/values.

Professional Differences and Consensus

One-way analyses of variance were performed to assess professional differences in ratings on each item and on each factor. Item-by-item comparisons yielded significant differences in mean professional ratings on 27 of 39 items. A comparison of mean professional ratings on each factor using one-way analysis of variance revealed significant differences on all factors except the physical abuse category. These findings are summarized in table B–4.

The predominant pattern of consensus in ratings was agreement between nurses and social workers, who rated items as significantly more serious than did pediatricians and psychiatrists. Psychologists were between these two extremes and did not differ significantly from the other groups. The exception to this pattern occurred for factor 2—parental sexual preference—to which nurses and pediatricians gave significantly higher seriousness ratings than did social workers.

With one exception, all professional groups were in agreement regarding rank ordering of seriousness of maltreatment categories. For psychiatrists, the "minor neglect/discipline" category was rated as more serious than "life-style/values."

Important Personal Variables

Sex Differences. Significant sex differences emerged on all factors except parental sexual preference, in *t*-test comparisons.[3] Since profession and sex were interrelated, sex differences were examined separately using *t*-tests within each professional group that contained enough members of each sex to analyze: social workers, pediatricians, and psychologists. No significant sex differences were found for social workers. In the psychologist and physician groups, one significant difference was found in each group. Female psychologists rated seriousness of general failures in care significantly higher than males. For physicians, females rated seriousness of physical abuse significantly higher than their male colleagues (table B–5).

Parenthood Status. A comparison of mean seriousness ratings of maltreatment categories for subjects who were or were not parents was performed. This was analyzed for the sample as a whole and

Table B–3

Categories Resulting from Exploratory Factor Analysis

Categories and Items	Loadings					
	I	II	III	IV	V	VI
I. General failures in care						
Child left alone at night; child starts fire	.74	.04	.20	.22	.04	.30
Child unwashed; covered with sores	.73	.10	.29	.19	.34	.04
Child severely emotionally disturbed; parents refuse treatment	.71	.02	.27	.11	.12	.19
Child not bathed; has impetigo	.71	.11	.21	.06	.46	.07
Child left out at night; wanders away from home	.70	.09	.07	.17	.08	.37
Child inadequately nourished; inadequate cooking facilities in home	.67	.11	.26	.19	.34	.10
Child kept home from school regularly, failing in school	.65	.18	.14	.00	.31	.36
Child on filthy mattress; has body sores	.65	.03	.27	.18	.33	.22
Parents dress son as a girl; child fights with others	.63	.09	.33	.16	.02	.25
Family lives in filthy, infested house	.63	.24	.18	.07	.40	.19
Child frequently truant; no action from parent	.62	.23	.20	.00	.28	.36
Parents use cocaine; child swallows laxatives	.60	.12	.11	.20	.11	.46
Child forced to overeat; health endangered	.59	.02	.04	.09	.38	.28
Parents drink with child; child becomes intoxicated	.58	.14	.18	.13	.26	.40
Parents ignore child's ear infection; inner ear damage follows	.58	.00	.18	.43	.35	.15
Child hospitalized 3 times for being underweight; gains in hospital	.57	.06	− .01	.21	.31	.32
Failure to give medication for throat infection	.52	.13	.00	.18	.45	.27
II. Parental sexual preference						
Child's father is a homosexual; child knows this	.12	.94	.07	.05	.14	.15
Child's mother is a lesbian; child knows this	.12	.93	.06	.03	.14	.16
III. Sexual abuse						
Sexual intercourse between child and parent; child has gonorrhea	.16	.07	.81	.07	.16	.05
Parent suggests to child that they have sex; child has nightmares	.30	.06	.74	.10	.08	.30
Parent and child engage in mutual masturbation; child makes sexual overtures to other children	.45	.02	.56	.26	.17	.22

Table B–3 continued

Categories and Items	Loadings					
	I	II	III	IV	V	VI
IV. Severe physical abuse						
Parent immerses child in hot water; child suffers burns	.20	.05	.19	.82	.11	.07
Parent bangs child against wall; child suffers concussion	.27	.04	.03	.79	.18	.18
V. Minor neglect/discipline						
Child runs around without clothes; has bad cold	.05	.21	.10	.20	.66	.10
Parent spanks the child; red marks on skin	.21	–.07	.11	.09	.63	.49
Failure to keep medical appointments; child has heart defect	.34	.04	.31	.17	.58	.07
VI. Life-style/values						
Parents make child take stolen goods to store; child knows they are stolen	.30	.15	.34	.08	.11	.66
Parent gets "high" smoking marijuana; child takes a drag	.34	.30	.07	.13	.22	.60
Parent spanks child with leather strap; red marks on skin	.35	–.02	.11	.20	.46	.57
Parents have intercourse and child sees them	.20	.11	.36	.09	.38	.55
Parent makes child steal from supermarket; child is caught[a]	.50	.21	.17	.11	.08	.54
Items Not Loading on Any Factor						
Parents ignore the child most of the time; child fights with others	.37	.08	.49	–.06	.37	.36
Parents do not make the child do his or her homework; child failing in school	.45	.27	.13	–.15	.45	.38
Family lives in old house; child cuts hand on broken glass	.47	.25	–.02	.17	.39	.40
Parents allow relative who is a prostitute to bring customers to house; child knows this	.36	.27	.32	.15	.08	.47
Parents feed only milk to child who has iron deficiency	.42	.16	.15	.06	.48	.08
Child wears filthy clothing	.44	.37	.11	.02	.49	.24

Note: Principal components factor analysis with Varimax rotation. These six factors accounted for 70% of the variance. The factor "general failures in care" accounted for 50% of the variance. A factor loading of .50 or better was used as a criterion for inclusion on a factor.

[a]This item also loaded on the factor "general failures in care."

Table B–4
Mean Seriousness Ratings of Factors by Profession

Category	Nurses	Social Workers	Psychologists	Physicians	Psychiatrists	F-value[a]
			Profession			
Physical abuse	8.61	8.55	8.45	8.29	8.57	1.42
Sexual abuse	8.41	8.42	8.25	8.10	7.82	2.84*
General failures in care	7.44	7.33	6.97	6.92	6.53	3.73**
Life-style/values	7.00	6.69	6.45	6.31	5.65	4.70***
Minor neglect/ discipline	6.53	6.66	6.41	5.85	5.89	4.14**
Parental sexual preference[b]	3.84	2.63	3.22	3.49	2.87	4.18*

Note: Groups sharing an underlining agree; groups differing in underlining differ significantly from each other.
[a]From one-way analyses of variance; a posteriori comparisons using Duncan's multiple range test.
[b]Social workers differed significantly from nurses and physicians on this category.
*$p < .05$; **$p < .01$; ***$p < .001$.

for each professional group, using *t*-tests. No significant difference according to parenthood status emerged for the sample as a whole. Within the social work and psychologist groups, however, significant differences were found for social workers in ratings of sexual abuse and life-style/values, and for psychologists in ratings of parental sexual preference. In cases where differences emerged, parents rated the category as significantly more serious than did nonparents (table B–6).

Years of Experience Posttraining. Correlations of years of experience by category seriousness ratings were performed for each professional group. A significant relationship was found only for nurses, occurring on all six factors. Years of experience correlated negatively with seriousness ratings on each factor (table B–7).

Prior Involvement with Cases of Child Abuse. This variable was not significantly related to seriousness ratings for any professional group.

Table B–5
*Significant Sex Differences in Mean Factor
Ratings within Professions*

Profession	Males		Females		t-values[a]
	M	SD	M	SD	
Psychologists					
General failures in care	6.14	1.51	7.29	1.13	2.28*
Minor neglect/ discipline	5.63	1.49	6.53	1.07	1.88[c]
n		8		24	
Physicians					
Physical abuse[b]	8.14	1.32	8.65	.61	2.36*
General failures in care	6.80	1.38	7.34	1.00	1.70[c]
n		55		23	

[a]From two-tailed *t*-tests.
[b]For this comparison, variances were significantly different and Satterthwaite's approximation was used.
[c]$p < .10$; *$p < .05$.

Table B–6
*Significant Differences by Parenthood Status
in Mean Factor Ratings within Professions*

Profession	Parent		Nonparent		t-values[a]
	M	SD	M	SD	
Social worker					
Sexual abuse[b]	8.64	.53	8.32	.77	2.22*
Life-style/values	7.16	1.24	6.48	1.37	2.17*
n		26		57	
Psychologists					
Parent sexual preference	4.45	2.48	2.66	1.57	2.49*
n		10		22	

[a]From two-tailed *t*-tests.
[b]For this comparison, variances were significantly different and Satterthwaite's approximation was used.
*$p < .05$.

Table B–7
*Correlation of Factor Seriousness Ratings with Years
of Experience for Nurses*

Category	Correlation Coefficient[a]
Physical abuse	− .33**
Sexual abuse	− .27**
General failures in care	− .36***
Life-style/values	− .42***
Minor neglect/discipline	− .30**
Parental sexual preference	− .22*

[a]Pearson's Rho.
*$p < .05$; **$p < .01$; ***$p < .001$.

Medical Specialty. A comparison of mean severity ratings of categories for three groups of physicians by medical specialty—medical students, pediatricians, and surgeons—indicated that surgeons rated seriousness lower on all categories than did the other doctors. These differences were significant for three categories: general failures in care, minor neglect, and life-style/values (table B–8).

Table B–8
*Mean Seriousness Ratings of Categories
by Medical Specialty*

Categories	Medical Students	Pediatricians	Surgeons	F-value[a]
Physical abuse	8.19	8.60	7.88	1.94
Sexual abuse	8.27	8.28	7.50	2.83[b]
General failures in care	7.10	7.14	6.05	3.68*
Life-style/values	6.39	6.67	5.18	4.98*
Minor neglect/discipline	6.06	6.17	4.47	6.31**
Parental sexual preference	3.42	3.77	3.38	.30

Note: Groups sharing an underlining agree. Groups differing in underlinings differ significantly from each other.
[a]One-way analyses of variance; a posteriori comparisons between means using Duncan's Multiple Range Test.
[b]$p < .10$; *$p < .05$; **$p < .01$.

Discussion

Defining Child Abuse:
Categories of Maltreatment

Results of this study suggest that professionals do discriminate among types of child maltreatment and are in some consensus regarding the relative seriousness of these categories for the welfare of the child. The failure to confirm the factor structure predicted based on the Giovannoni and Becerra study findings is not surprising, given the differences between the two studies. The current study uses only half the number of vignette items (39 of 78). In addition, Giovannoni and Becerra's sample included only one hospital-based group of professionals, pediatricians, whereas the present study was designed to assess seriousness ratings by medical and mental health professionals in a hospital setting.

While fewer factors emerged in this study, three of the six factors are conceptually similar to factors in the Giovannoni and Becerra analysis. These are: physical abuse, sexual abuse, and general failures in care. Some categories which emerged as separate factors in the Giovannoni and Becerra study were subsumed under the "general failures in care" factor in this study. The two weakest factors in this study—minor neglect/discipline, and life-style/values—did not have conceptual parallels among the Giovannoni and Becerra factors, but included items which loaded on a number of different factors in their study (e.g., failure to provide; fostering delinquency, drugs, and alcohol; sexual mores) or did not load on any factors in their study (e.g., the spanking item).

Each of these two factors in the current study included items representing a variety of caretaking situations. For the life-style/values factor, the similarity among constituent items is one of life-style or moral deviance from the cultural norm: fostering criminal behavior, use of drugs, and open sexual behavior. The exception is the spanking item, which conceptually would seem to fit with the "minor neglect/discipline" items. Spanking, however, is controversial, being socially acceptable to some groups and unacceptable to others (e.g., Erlanger, 1975; "The Last? Resort," 1985; Straus, Gelles & Steinmetz, 1980). Thus, use of corporal punishment may be considered a life-style difference, although it differs from other items found in this category.

Among the "minor neglect/discipline" items, the commonality appears to be in the domain of physical care, but with less serious consequences for the child than for items loading on "general failures in care."

The "parental sexual preference" factor in this study emerged as a conceptually distinct category, not loading with other life-style items. (In the Giovannoni and Becerra analysis, these items loaded with other "sexual more" items not included in this study.) This category was also rated as least serious for the welfare of the child. The mean rating for the entire sample was 3.29, a full 3 points below the next highest category and in the "not at all serious" range. These findings strongly suggest that parental sexual preference does not belong in the domain of child maltreatment.

Differences among Professional Groups

Similar to the findings of earlier studies (Gelles, 1975; Turbett & O'Toole, 1980), consensus within this study was greatest on the severe physical abuse items, where the maltreatment appeared intentional and resulted in physical harm to the child.

The consistent patterns of agreement and disagreement among professional groups (in mean ratings of other categories of maltreatment, as well as of individual items) point to differences in training and work roles. This may reflect the fact that nurses and social workers tended to rate vignettes and categories at the high end of the seriousness scale. These two professions are the "front line" for inpatient cases in which there is a question of maltreatment. Nurses have the most frequent contact with the child, as well as ongoing contact with parents. Social workers are in contact with parents, attempting to forge a relationship and to complete an assessment. The training of both professions heavily emphasizes social and psychological factors in child and family functioning, thereby increasing sensitivity to more subtle kinds of child maltreatment and potential consequences. The observations nurses and social workers make are usually critical in decision making about the filing of child abuse reports. Hence, the burden of recognition may fall heavily on their shoulders.

One would expect psychologists and psychiatrists to have training emphasis similar to that of nurses and social workers, and to
be sensitive to social and psychological circumstances as well; yet
psychiatrists consistently rated incidents as less serious than any
other group, with physicians next lowest, preceded by psychologists
(table B–4). Psychologists and psychiatrists are involved with possible cases of child maltreatment in two ways: as diagnostic consultants on inpatient cases, and as ongoing therapists. In the former
role they have fleeting contact, often a single interview with patient and parents, or perhaps no contact with parents at all. While
their observations are important, their temporal and emotional
involvement is limited. In their role as therapists, their focus is
primarily on potential long-term effects and on preventive intervention. In the vignettes, however, consequences to the child were situational and immediate. Long-term consequences had to be inferred
by the reader. It is possible that psychologists and psychiatrists,
trained to ameliorate long term psychological damage, may deem
phasize the "harm" produced from isolated incidents or parenting
mishaps. Their training embodies the belief that intervention can
ameliorate psychological damage and that single incidents do not
in themselves produce irreversible harm.

The relatively lower seriousness ratings by physicians, who
would be expected to have daily contact with hospitalized patients
and to have the prime role in case management, is probably best
explained by their biomedical as opposed to psychosocial orientation. This focus emphasizes physical symptomatology to the ex-
clusion of psychological difficulties. In addition, physician involvement with the patient and family, though frequent, is more fleeting
than that of nurses and social workers. Physicians' relatively low
ratings compared to nurses and social workers parallels their place
in the rankings by professional groups in the Giovannoni and
Becerra study.

Further analysis within the physician group by specialty revealed
a consistent pattern of significant differences in mean seriousness
ratings. This supports the notion that training and work role effect evaluation of seriousness. Surgeons consistently rated categories
as less serious than medical students or pediatricians (significantly
so in areas of minor neglect and life-style/values, and approaching
significance for sexual abuse). The focus of surgeons is even more

"biomedical" and less holistic than is true for pediatricians and medical students, and their contact with parents is apt to be minimal.

Caution must be raised in considering the implications of these professional differences. How the ratings relate to actual *behavior* in clinical decision making cannot be determined from this study. However, a 3-month review of contacts by hospital professionals with the child abuse consulting team and observation of the team's weekly update meeting indicate that there may be some behavioral correlates to the response tendencies found in this study.[4] Social workers are most likely to refer cases to the team for consultation. Pediatricians were the second most likely group to refer. In many cases, however, the latter group reported reluctantly, after prodding from social workers and nurses. Contacts from psychologists and psychiatrists to the team were quite infrequent. A more systematic study of hospital practices in recognition and management of possible child maltreatment cases, through review of case records and reports filed, could shed more light on the association between the attitudes reflected in this study and actual behavior.

A second caution in drawing implications about professional differences from the current study stems from examining the absolute differences between group means. While differences are significant, they are small in actual magnitude, and ratings tend to be within the same range of seriousness. Hence, there appears to be a good deal of *agreement* among the professional groups.

Personal Variables and Seriousness Ratings

Differences in factor ratings across professional groups by the personal variables of parenthood status, years of experience, and prior involvement with child abuse cases were not significant. Sex differences were significant on all categories except parental sexual preference, but sex was confounded with profession. Personal variables were also examined within professional groups. Women rated incidents as more serious than men, and parents gave higher ratings than did nonparents. The correlation between number of years of experience in one's profession with seriousness ratings of maltreatment categories was significant only for nurses, and the relationship was negative. Perhaps this reflects a generational difference, or a desensitization effect related to many years of inpatient experience. Thus, *profession appears to be the variable that best accounts for rating differences.*

Conclusions

A number of conclusions can be drawn from the findings of this study.

1. Hospital professionals discriminate among child maltreatment categories and agree on the rank ordering of their seriousness for the welfare of the child.

In conjunction with Giovannoni and Becerra's (1979) findings, this suggests that definitions of child maltreatment used in clinical practice, state reporting laws, and research studies could be made more precise. Clear guidelines for practice according to maltreatment category might be developed by specifying circumstances meriting intervention.

2. Parental sexual preference does not belong in the domain of child maltreatment.

Professionals were in agreement in assigning ratings at the "nonserious" end of the scale to this category. Parental sexual preference was distinct from other life-style items and should not be grounds for protective intervention.

3. Significant differences in seriousness ratings by profession occurred in all categories except severe physical abuse.

These differences are best accounted for by work roles and training. Frontline nurses and social workers give the highest seriousness ratings, and psychiatrists give significantly lower ratings. Whether these differences reflect a difference in response tendency or a difference apparent from the level of professional involvement cannot be determined from this study.

4. Despite differences found among professionals in ratings of seriousness, there was also much consensus.

The absolute differences in mean ratings were generally small. The ranking of maltreatment categories by seriousness was almost identical. Hence, the emphasis must be on consensus among hospital professionals in evaluating incidents of child maltreatment.

Further study should focus on differences and similarities in behavior among professionals when recognizing and responding to cases of possible child maltreatment, as well as analyzing the relationship between attitudes and behavior. Behavioral differences could be examined indirectly through case record review or more directly through observation of actual practice. Correlations between attitudes and behavior might be examined in a variety of ways. For example, in addition to rating seriousness of incidents for the welfare of a child, professionals might be asked to indicate what action should be taken. Finally, it would be useful to systematically investigate what specific information effects the evaluation of seriousness by different disciplines (e.g., nature of the consequence, parental characteristics, child characteristics, family socioeconomic status, ethnic group). Understanding interdisciplinary differences and similarities in attitudes and behavior in these cases would facilitate better communication among professionals, and improve clinical practice.

Notes

1. In the 1983 national statistics of reported child abuse cases (AHA, 1983), only 3.2% involved a "major physical injury," 18.5% involved "minor physical injury," and 5.2% involved an injury of unspecified severity. The most commonly reported type of maltreatment is "deprivation of necessities." The less obvious case may well be the norm.
2. Physicians' level of training:

	Medical students	Residents	Postresidency
Number of physicians	32	21	25

3. When variances between groups were significantly different, Satterthwaite's approximation was used.
4. Boston Children's Hospital interdisciplinary child abuse team has been operating since 1970. At the time of this study it was composed of two social workers, a psychiatrist, a psychologist, a nurse, a pediatrician, and a hospital attorney. The team acts as a consulting group and becomes active only when a case is referred to them for review and advice on case management, including whether to file a report to the state protective service agency. Most referrals to the team are inpatient cases. On most hospital divisions, any of the involved professionals can refer a case to the team; on some, the referral has to come from the physician in charge of the case.

References

American Humane Association (1983). Annual Report. *Highlights of official child neglect and abuse reporting.* Denver, CO.

Bourne, R. & Newberger, E.H. (1980). Interdisciplinary process group in the hospital management of child abuse and neglect. *Child Abuse and Neglect,* 4, 137–144.

Daniel, J.H. (1985). Cultural and ethnic issues: The black family. In E.H. Newberger and R. Bourne (Eds.), *Unhappy families: Clinical and research perspectives on family violence* (pp. 145–154). Littleton, MA: Publishing Sciences Group.

Elmer, E. (1960). Abused young children seen in hospitals. *Social Work, 5,* 98–102.

Erlanger, H.S. (1975). Social class differences in parents' use of physical punishment. In S.K. Steinmetz and M.A. Straus (Eds.), *Violence in the family.* New York: Dodd, Mead & Co.

Gelles, R.J. (1973). Child abuse as psychopathology: A sociological critique and reformulation. *American Journal of Orthopsychiatry, 43,* 611–621.

Gelles, R.J. (1975). Community agencies and child abuse: Labelling and gatekeeping. Paper presented at the Conference on Recent Research on the Family, sponsored by the Society for Research in Child Development, Ann Arbor, MI.

Giovannoni, J.M., & Becerra, R.M. (1979). *Defining child abuse.* New York: Free Press.

Hampton, R.L. & Newberger, E.H. (1985). Child abuse incidence and reporting by hospitals: Significance of severity, class, and race. *American Journal of Public Health, 75,* 56–60.

Helfer, R.E. (1975). Why most physicians don't get involved in child abuse and what to do about it. *Children Today, 4,* 28–31.

Hill, D.A. (1975). Emotional reaction to child abuse within a hospital setting. In N.B. Ebeling and D.A. Hill (Eds.), *Child abuse: Intervention and treatment.* Acton, MA: Publishing Sciences Group.

Katz, M., Hampton, R., Newberger, E., Bowles, R., & Snyder, J. (1986). Returning children home: Clinical decision making in cases of child abuse and neglect. *American Journal of Orthopsychiatry, 56,* 253–262.

Kaufman, I. (1983). The professional use of the self: Transference and counter-transference. In N.B. Ebeling and D.A. Hill (Eds.), *Child abuse and neglect.* Littleton, MA: Publishing Sciences Group.

Korbin, J. (1977). Anthropological contributions to the study of child abuse. *Child Abuse and Neglect, 1,* 7–24.

"The Last? Resort" (1985). *Newsletter of the Committee to End Violence against the Next Generation, Inc. 14.*

Nagi, S.Z. (1977). *Child maltreatment in the United States.* New York: Columbia University Press.

Nalepka, C., O'Toole, R., & Turbett, J.P. (1981). Nurses and physicians' recognition and reporting of child abuse. *Comprehensive Pediatric Nursing, 5,* 33–38.

Newberger, E.H., Rosenfeld, A.A., Hyde, J.N., & Holter, J.C. (1978). Child abuse and child neglect. In R.A. Hoekelman, S. Blauman, P.A. Brunell, S.B. Friedman, & H.M. Seidel (Eds.), *Principles of pediatrics: Health care of the young.* New York: McGraw-Hill.

Rosenfeld, A.A. & Newberger, E.H. (1977). Compassion vs. control: Conceptual and practical pitfalls in the broadened definition of child abuse. *Journal of the American Medical Association, 237,* 2086–2088.

Rosenzweig, H.D. (1982). Some considerations in the management of child abuse: A psychiatric consultant's perspective. In E.H. Newberger (Ed.), *Child abuse.* Boston: Little Brown.

Rosenzweig, H.D. (1985). Psychiatric issues and the physician's role in reporting child abuse. In E.H. Newberger and R. Bourne (Eds.), *Unhappy families: Clinical and research perspectives on family violence.* Littleton, MA: Publishing Sciences Group.

Straus, M., Gelles, R., & Steinmetz, S. (1980). *Behind closed doors: Violence in the American family.* Garden City: Anchor/Doubleday.

Turbett, J.P., & O'Toole, R. (1980). Physicians' recognition of child abuse. Paper presented at the Annual Meeting of the American Sociological Association, New York, N.Y.

Reprints: Requests for reprints should be sent to Eli H. Newberger, M.D., Director, Family Development Program, Children's Hospital, 300 Longwood Ave., Boston, MA 02115.

Appendix C
Interdisciplinary Group Process in the Hospital Management of Child Abuse and Neglect

Richard Bourne, J.D., Ph.D.
Eli H. Newberger, M.D.

The group process aspects of child protection in a children's hospital are examined. A team approach to case management enables personal support for individual members experiencing the strong emotions attached to protective service cases, eases the burden of individual decision making, and divides the complex tasks of data gathering and analysis. Confusion is fostered by inattention to personal and group expectations, individual roles, the status structure, and the methods for maintaining social cohesion. A team handbook may help to standardize decision making, but in such efforts to reduce conflict, group norms may be obscured. Task-oriented and social-emotional norms are discussed, and guidelines are offered to foster a more adequate approach to group problem solving.

This work originally appeared in *Child Abuse and Neglect* 4:137–144, 1980. Copyright © 1980 Pergamon Press. Reprinted with permission.

Introduction

Although the purpose of this paper is to discuss some of the management problems of multidisciplinary child abuse teams, we would first like to comment more generally on the present state of child protection.

These are troubled times for those concerned with the protection of children. Fifteen years after the promulgation of a model child abuse reporting law by the Children's Bureau, a law which was adopted in principle and subsequently broadened by every state, we are struggling to come to terms with a near deluge of reported cases of child abuse and neglect.

Not only are scarce child welfare resources strained to meet the enormous demand, but also the very ability of child protective services to address the needs of troubled families is increasingly brought into question.

Concern for the Quality of Protective Service Practice

The steady expansion of the definitions of child abuse and neglect in state reporting laws, for example, is sharply questioned in the draft child protection standard of the American Bar Association's Juvenile Justice Standards Project. The underlying premise of this volume of the Project, which we have addressed elsewhere [1], is that the sanctity of the family must be preserved from the blundering efforts of state social workers. The basis for juvenile court jurisdiction is narrowed too in this model legislation, which would, in addition, make the professional reporting of child neglect discretionary rather than mandatory.

Further criticism of the quality of protective service practice appears in the initial volume of the report of the Carnegie Council on Children, 1977.

After questioning not only the competency but the good faith of child welfare workers, the Commission endorses the findings and recommendations of the Juvenile Justice Standards Project. To quote from its report:

Large numbers of American families frequently find themselves in economic and emotional distress. Whether they are victims of chronic fatigue or of a crisis ranging from unemployment, not enough money, and depressing living conditions to physical disabilities, alcoholism, or mental illness, most of these families could be significantly helped by very practical aids such as more money, better housing, homemaking assistance, employment counseling or training, or temporary respite from the children in day-care programs. Sometimes they may need family counseling or individual treatment of the parent. But the parents in these families are not necessarily unfit; they are often responding to tremendous pressures. All too often, an arrogant state legal apparatus invokes the doctrine that the parents are "neglecting" their children and removes the children without attempting to give the family the supportive help it needs—for example, the money to buy food, pay the rent, or pay the homemaker who could care temporarily for the children while the parent recuperates from illness or goes out to look for a job. Even conscientious social workers and court personnel often have no power to command the tangible resources that might help the family continue intact. All they have is the coarsest implement: removal of the child.

This means that well-intentioned and even not-so-well-intentioned courts and social workers, acting in the "best interests of the child," can impose their norms of morality and upbringing upon families. Families live differently from one another, they treat children differently, they expect different standards of behavior, and they punish differently. Most families accused of abuse and neglect are minority families with low incomes, often one-parent families. Judges and court personnel, on the other hand, generally come from quite another social, economic, and ideological world. Behavior that may be quite normal in another social milieu may be shocking to them in terms of their own, and as a result they can be too quick to condemn and not eager enough to invest time and attention in trying to help [2].

Workers in the child protection field must take these comments seriously. At the least, they will partially discredit child welfare work. This discrediting, in turn, may lead to even fewer resources being appropriated by state legislatures.

To come to terms with this serious challenge to child welfare work, we urge workers in the field critically to scrutinize their practice.

Our own work convinces us of the strength of an interdisciplinary approach to child protection, and we offer the following critical analysis of the group process aspects of child protection in a children's hospital. We examine group process with the goal of recommending improvements in Trauma X Team functioning.

Group Processes

The Trauma X Group

The Trauma X Group at Children's Hospital Medical Center is an interdisciplinary team consisting of a pediatrician, attorney, psychiatric social worker, psychologist, nurse, and occasional other consultants, all of whom assist in the management of child abuse and neglect cases seen within the institution. The Group was organized in 1970. Since its inception, it has served to focus attention on child abuse and neglect at Children's Hospital, and an early evaluation suggested its effectiveness in promoting case management and in lessening reinjury [3].

When considering the formation of an interdisciplinary team, a crucial issue is the advantage of team structure as opposed to individual management and decision making. If tasks can be performed by one person working alone, then group involvement is unnecessary.

Group Dynamics Theory

Group dynamics theory gives a framework for understanding both positive and negative aspects of a team approach. In general, two principles maintain:

1. For tasks which involve creating ideas or remembering information, there is a greater possibility that one of several persons will find a good solution or produce information than will a single individual [4].

2. When several individuals work collectively on a single task, a division of labor is possible. This division of labor allows individuals to perform the tasks for which they are most qualified; prevents or reduces overlapping activity; and allows decisions to be made more rapidly than would occur were one person responsible for gathering data from a variety of sources or specializations. Protective service work lends itself to such task division.

Child abuse and neglect involve many specialities, each of which has differing and unique definitions of the situation presented. If, for example, a child enters the emergency ward with a fracture, the physician might determine whether the nature of the break indicates inflicted trauma; the social worker would interview the child's parents in order to evaluate their capacity to protect the child and to form a relationship on which might be based a program to prevent the injury from reoccurring; and the attorney might consider the desirability of a restraining order to prevent removal of the child from the hospital prior to a full assessment. The primary rationale for an interdisciplinary team, then, is that many skills are required for effective task performance.

A team approach, moreover, has other functions or advantages specifically in regard to child abuse and neglect. *First*, these problems stimulate strong emotional reactions in all of us: anger, sadness, and frustration are all too familiar. If group management exists, members can support one another and allay some of the personal distress inevitably associated with tragedy. *Second*, decision making in this area affects family welfare and the safety and health of children. It is easier for a group to bear the consequences of its decisions than for an individual alone to select, and live with, his or her recommendations. *Third*, abuse and neglect cases are complex and take much time and effort to resolve. A team is able to divide the labor in such a way that outcomes are facilitated.

Team management, on the other hand, may make for confusion and conflict unless the following issues are resolved:

1. What are the norms of group practice? (I.e., what expectations or "rules" exist within the group?) In order for a group to

function effectively, there must be consensus about what rules apply to the group and to individual participants. For example, all members might agree that everyone need participate in decisions concerning case disposition (this is consensus on a group norm), but that levels of participation might differ according to the nature of the decision, the personality of the participant, and the member's status and expertise (this is consensus on individual norms within the group).

2. What roles do individuals play? By the word "role" we mean not merely professional identification, but form of participation: asking questions or giving opinions, increasing solidarity or showing disagreement.

3. What is the status structure? In a hospital setting physicians usually have the greatest authority or influence. Groups in general might emphasize collegiality or hierarchy depending upon their task.

4. How is social cohesion maintained? In the interdisciplinary team, multiple divisions exist which potentially disrupt group unity and harm morale: differing professional orientations and commitments; ideological variations [5]; diverse interpersonal styles; race and social class distinctions.

Problems Implicit in Interdisciplinary Practice

Interdisciplinary teams, moreover, create problems which may decrease effectiveness:

1. When an expert maintains influence outside his own areas of expert knowledge. An example might be a hospital setting where a physician, because of high status, has his or her assessment of family dynamics accepted merely because no group member dares to question authority.

2. When a group member conforms in order to buy social approval. To take a position different from one's colleagues may invite rejection; it may be easier to conform to the opinions or evaluations of the other participants.

3. When the responsible person is unwilling to assume the risks involved in making a decision himself, problems are often referred

to committees for decision [6]. The group process would be a diffusion or spreading of responsibility, resulting in an increased tendency to risk taking.

This result has both positive and negative aspects: it allows action to be taken when fear of consequences might be inhibiting; on the other hand, it allows single individuals to escape full responsibility for ineffective or damaging intervention.

An example of the positive aspect is a case in which a child was brought to the Hospital with severe skull fractures. The parents were affluent and had much influence in their community. When confronted with an evaluation that the injury was inflicted, they denied both neglect and abuse and threatened suit if the case were pursued. Team management not only made the data base more reliable and valid (e.g., by producing medical and social indices of abuse) but also allowed decisions to be presented to parents as a group consensus an evaluation that was more difficult to confront, rebut, or alter than would be a recommendation by a single staffer.

An example of the negative is when everyone's business becomes no one's responsibility. Accountability under such a system is impossible.

4. Cases, or individual responses to cases, become routinized. Professionals who have worked in child protection know how easy it is to confuse cases (mixing the facts of one abuse incident, for example, with that of another). It is equally common to fall into group or individual patterns so that certain types of cases are managed similarly despite differences in facts. For example, the team might have conferred on cases where addicted mothers neglected or abused their children; each time an "addicted mother" case appears, the same recommendations may be made despite differences in type or degree of addiction, family supports, impact of mother's addiction on her charge, etc. Or, for example, a social worker might have seen one of her cases successfully resolved through the court process; in most subsequent decision making, court to her becomes a preferred alternative. Such patterns, reinforced by group norms, must be avoided in order that each problem

be treated sensitively and individually. It is an unending challenge to think each case through anew, instead of responding automatically once certain information is communicated (e.g., mother must have abused her child because mother herself was abused when she was a child).

5. Group members, and other hospital staffers, become so accustomed to depending on others that they do not think and learn on their own. When a legal problem arises, for example, the lawyer is automatically consulted—because he might be offended were someone else to enter his turf or because it is safer to share decision making. Such discussion occurs even when the same or very similar issues have been discussed before; individuals do not expand their expertise, and time is wasted.

6. Team members do not understand group process. An understanding of group process is not inborn but arises from learning and experience. It is important, therefore, that members become aware of such process, probably through the use of a group's expert. An example of misunderstanding might be the attribution of group "problems" to personality factors (e.g., "we don't like one another . . . that's why the team isn't effective") instead of a more sociologically based analysis (intermember conflict is symptomatic of differences over group goals or objectives).

7. Intelligent problem solving is limited by the fact that different disciplines view the same data in different ways and that, across disciplines, there is an inability to understand the concepts and tools of other specializations. Each profession is oriented to specific ethics, goals, and methods of practice.

For example, a sociologist analyzing the causes of abuse would look to the social context in which the behavior occurs—the strains or pressures that triggered aggression. A psychologist, on the other hand, might focus on the individual perpetrator. Examining past experiences as a predictor of present action he would ask, "What sort of a person would act in this way?" and would attempt to construct a psychological type from developmental history and from attitudinal/behavioral data. To a psychologist social context is often the circumstance precipitating violence, not the primary cause of such; the violence, defined as endemic, was probably inevitable despite the chance stimulus which induced it.

A lawyer, moreover, would probably belittle the sociologist's conception of social forces pressuring behavior; he might also reject the common psychological orientation that the human being is irrationally motivated by unconscious forces and drives established in infancy or early childhood. To a lawyer a person might be viewed as rationally able to choose among alternatives; possessing "free will," the person chooses to commit a criminal act (unless legally insane) and must bear the legal and social consequences of his behavior.

The legal perspective also may differ from that of the physician and social worker. Though interested in treatment of the violence-prone, the lawyer accepts the need for punishment: the criminal is a wrongdoer who is responsible for his deviance, not a victim exculpated by forces beyond control.

Norms, Roles, and Status Structure in Shaping Conflict and Consensus

After observing the Children's Hospital trauma team and its interaction patterns, we believe that the press for social cohesion is a most important determinant of its functioning.

Though the team's norms, for the most part, are not codified, there is a handbook written by the group which outlines the tasks each participant is to perform. It also attempts to standardize decision making by indicating when various procedures are appropriate (e.g., the taking of a trauma case to court). This handbook is felt important because it educates members and lessens arbitrariness, but a latent function is the reduction of conflict. We attempt to use guidelines to avoid differences of opinion and to resolve those differences which do arise.

Information on child abuse, if shared, is another basis of team consensus. If all members agree that "a mother who was abused is more likely to abuse," then decision making is simplified and group unity facilitated. Except for group benefits it apparently matters little that some of this commonly accepted information is untrue, only occasionally accurate, or simplistic [7].

Norms. Group norms also encourage cohesion and harmony. They might be divided into two categories: the task-oriented and the social-emotional. The task emphasis is on consensus decision making; that is, all participants should agree with a particular course of action. If strong differences do occur, especially as between the medical and social work perspectives, nothing is done until they are resolved. Social-emotional norms include the following: don't lose one's temper in disagreement (disagreement should be resolved through rational discussion); and members should be supportive of one another (by showing solidarity).

Task norm. The following cases illustrate how group unity is maintained through consensus decision making.

In the first case, a child was brought into the Children's Hospital emergency ward; black and blue marks were scattered across his body with no particular pattern. His mother reported that in the past such marks had spontaneously appeared and, after a few days' time, had gradually faded. Medical staff suspected inflicted injury, a suspicion which grew after testing failed to detect any organic basis for the discoloration. A social worker met with the parents, who seemed appropriate and apparently lacked the characteristics associated with abusers (i.e., they were not socially isolated, they did not hold unrealistic expectations for their son, etc.). The parents denied ever having left the child with another caretaker.

The trauma team met to confer on the case, and medical and social service staff were strongly divided as to the nature of the problem and the preferred disposition: the first group urged court as a means of conducting a more thorough evaluation of the family, while the second felt any action would be unjustified as the failure to find a medical explanation did not exclude its possibility. After much discussion the group decided to file a mandatory report to the Department of Public Welfare, a middle course which reconciled and satisfied all participants.

In a second case, a child residing in another state was admitted to the Hospital for back surgery. Staff nurses noticed that the patient seemed depressed and urged a psychiatric consultation. This evaluation revealed not only depression but also self-destructive tendencies, most of which seemingly originated from a disturbed relationship with her parents. The child reported, for example, that for the past several years she had been sexually abused by her father with the passive acceptance of her mother; that her father had been physically violent to both her and her mother; and that a protective action had been initiated on these grounds in family court of the state of residence.

The team was conflicted over the appropriate alternative. One member argued that because the child was in our institution we had an obligation to protect her; that such protection (and the concomitant services and supports) was surer in Massachusetts courts and facilities than in those out-of-state; that under no circumstances could she be discharged home; and that the preferred disposition would be the initiation of a care and protection petition in Massachusetts if parents were uncooperative toward the recommendation of residential psychiatric placement. A second member, on the other hand, argued that since the family lived out-of-state, since our involvement with the child had been brief, and since out-of-state authorities were aware of and had taken action to resolve the problem, that we, after informing these authorities of our findings, should essentially adopt a "hands off" position. Indeed, as between discharging the child home and initiating a Massachusetts petition, the former was preferable as the girl's parents could not easily receive therapy (or be involved in their daughter's treatment) so far from home. Massachusetts, moreover, would likely be unwilling to provide service to (spend money on) out-of-staters despite its obligation to do so if it accepted jurisdiction of the case and legal custody of the minor.

As these competing positions seemed impossible to reconcile, the hospital administration was called upon to determine the nature and extent of team involvement. That is, when consensus was not reached, the administration acted as a mediator, resolving the dispute in a way that was agreeable to all and, thus, lessening the likelihood of a protracted difference of opinion which would undercut group unity.

Admittedly, it is easier to arrive at a valid decision if medical and social data are corroborative. In those cases where the different disciplines lead to different conclusions, however, not only is case management less confidently conducted but also the team is strained and cohesion undermined. Therefore, a tendency exists to: (*a*) reach a compromise acceptable to all; (*b*) make no decision until further data clearly make one position more credible; (*c*) allow the decision to be made by an "impartial" arbiter.

The importance of consensus orientation is its impact on families. If a decision is reached because it flows from the facts of a case, then intervention can be rationally justified. But if a decision is made, not because of case data but because of team dynamics and group unity, then it might assist the team to the detriment of parents and children alike.

Social-Emotional Norm. The social support norm is functional because of the stress of decision making in trauma cases: a child improperly discharged home might return to the hospital reinjured while a decision to remove a child from biological parents obviously has much impact on a family and on those who must determine the child's "best interests."

Social support is also important because of the way the team is defined within the hospital setting. Generally hospital staff do not like trauma cases: they are complex, unpleasant, and demanding. Though the team is supposedly a consultative group, moreover, it is frequently seen as "taking over" from the treating physicians (e.g., when discharge is delayed because of family conditions despite the fact that the child is medically ready to depart); it is not clear, that is, what decisions belong to the team and how authority should be divided between the team and other hospital professional staff.

These two factors—nature of the cases and unclear relationships with personnel—strain communications and feelings between the team and others and make it more important for trauma members to support their colleagues. The more hostile the external environment becomes, in fact, the more cohesive do the members of the team seemingly become. Group cohesion is sometimes increased by this we/they orientation which implies that foolish decisions are made by others in the hospital (e.g., orthopedists mending a bone think that such treatment alone is sufficient to aid an abused child). This orientation stems from a legitimate concern that the needs of children and families are being slighted but also from a fear that our expertise is going unrecognized or that lack of consultations will threaten team survival (by showing that our input is unnecessary to effective case management—or will be so perceived). In a sense, we must emphasize our own worth because we are operating in an environment too willing to dismiss us and our role.

Conferring on cases also fosters group cohesion. Individual members meet together and the meeting itself reaffirms team existence.

It must be added that conflict among team members is not necessarily destructive or dysfunctional for the group [8]. A lack of conflict, indeed, might indicate that the team structure is so fragile that no one would risk confrontation because of a fear of dissolution. If disagreements are hidden or remain unresolved, then hostility builds up in such a way that the slightest difference can spark sudden and intense rupture.

In our experience, how conflicts are handled, not their existence, is the more appropriate focus. Goffman distinguishes "backstage" from "frontstage" [9]—in this context, between team disagreement which is private and that which is public. Private divisions of opinion are healthy and lead to the education of individual group members as well as to more effective decision making. Public disagreement, on the other hand, may embarrass participants and confuse those who desire and request consultation and input. If there is much interpersonal and interdisciplinary conflict, however, the quality of group decisions might lessen, task effectiveness being partially dependent on the relationship among team members.

Roles. After operating in an interdisciplinary setting for a period of time, the different participants become comfortable with the language and thought processes of the various specialties. The pediatrician, for example, might venture a psychiatric assessment, or the social worker a legal analysis. This crossing of disciplines, however, is usually done with the realization that turf is being violated: apologies are given ("I don't mean to get into your area"), statements qualified ("I'm no lawyer, but . . ."), or immediate deference shown if the nonexpert statement is challenged by the authority. In this way, members feel sufficiently free to transcend their narrow roles but not so as to threaten or question the capacity of their associates.

Implicit in decision making is the feeling that the person with the most firsthand information should play a pivotal role; that the opinions of outside staff should be respected, if not accepted (otherwise the team will not be voluntarily consulted on future cases); that participation should come from all members; that those who have seen the child and/or family describe, while the rest either question or suggest; that the lawyer is the skeptic, probing conclusions (e.g., "the parents are disorganized," "mother is crazy") and emphasizing the need for objective data.

Status. Despite the fact that in the larger society, and in the hospital, a physician has greater status than a nurse or social worker, the team operates under a norm of collegiality, i.e., that all disciplines are equally important in decision making; that the quality and logic of a suggestion is more important than the person offering it; that no person or role has the right to veto a recommendation acceptable to other group members. This norm, too, increases individual assertiveness and the feeling that one may operate without fear of sanction—all of which leads to group morale, commitment, and cohesion. Task effectiveness is likewise enhanced as no single discipline has greater knowledge or insight into child abuse management, and thus no single discipline should be accorded weight merely because of what it is as opposed to what it contributes.

One of the ways to share power is to rotate the conference chairperson rather than having the same discussion leader at each meeting. This device of course might merely disguise the true power structure, but if used properly it can enhance team collegiality.

Conclusion

Guidelines for More Effective Interdisciplinary Practice

We conclude with the following recommendations to foster a more nearly adequate approach to group problem solving and practice in child protection work:

1. Promote understanding of group process in professionals of each discipline.

2. Enable communication and conflict both individually, between members, and in the larger group context by structuring sufficient private time for the members of the group to use to promote cohesion.

3. Develop group consensus on leadership style and the flow of decisions. (Our preference is for a collective and interactive, as opposed to a hierarchical, model of organization, with each discipline on an equal footing.)

4. Identify in all conferences—at the outset—decision points to be reached, and to the extent possible enable discussion of their consequences, for child, for family, and for professionals. At the end of each conference decisions made should be explicitly stated so as to avoid misunderstandings among participants.

5. Enable expression, at conferences, of each discipline's perspective on the available data. This can be facilitated by rotating the chairing of the meeting among disciplines, with the person from the group most knowledgeable on a particular case assuming the leadership role.

References

1. Bourne, R., and Newberger, E., "Family autonomy" vs "Coercive intervention"?: Ambiguity and conflict in a proposed juvenile justice standard on child protection. *Boston U. Law Rev.* 57(4):670–706 (1977).
2. Kenniston, K., and the Carnegie Council on Children. All our children. *The American Family under Pressure.* Harcourt Brace Jovanovich, New York (1977), pp. 186–187.
3. Newberger, E., et al., Reducing the literal and human cost of child abuse: Impact of a new hospital management system. *Pediat.* 51(5):840–848 (1973).
4. Collins, B., and Guetzkow, H., *A Social Psychology of Group Processes for Decision-Making.* Wiley, New York (1964), p. 20.
5. Rosenfeld, A., and Newberger, E., Compassion vs control: Conceptual and practical pitfalls in the broadened definition of child abuse. *J. Amer. Med. Assoc.* 237:2086–2088 (1977).

6. Marquis, D.G., Individual responsibility and group decision involving risk. *Indust. Manage. Rev.* 3 (1962).
7. Gelles, R., Violence towards children in the United States. *Am. J. Orthopschiat.* 48:580–592. The estimates of the prevalence of family violence which can be drawn from this study suggest that there are many more child and adult victims of abuse than previously believed; the data impel reexamination of the common wisdoms which are based on studies of small samples of "caught" cases. We have compiled a series of essays which challenge existing assumptions in the protective service field in Bourne, R., and Newberger, E. (eds.), *Critical Perspectives on Child Abuse.* Lexington Books, Lexington, Mass. (1979).
8. Coser, L. *The Functions of Social Conflict.* Free Press, Glencoe, Ill. (1956).
9. Goffman, E., *The Presentation of Self in Everyday Life.* Doubleday, Garden City, N.Y. (1959).

Appendix D
Returning Children Home:
Clinical Decision Making in Cases
of Child Abuse and Neglect

Mitchell H. Katz, B.A.
Robert L. Hampton, Ph.D.
Eli H. Newberger, M.D.
Roy T. Bowles, Ph.D.
Jane C. Snyder, Ph.D.

Factors that influence the decision to remove children from their parents'
care in cases of abuse and neglect were examined by reviewing hospital
records of 185 children. Children with physical injuries were more likely
to be placed in a foster home or in residential care if they were from
poor families, while those with nonphysical injuries were more likely
to be removed if their families were more affluent. Implications for clinical
decision making are considered.

Cases of child abuse and neglect confront clinicians with the difficult practical and ethical dilemma of whether to initiate action
to remove children from their parents' care. On the one hand, the
doctrine to "above all else, do no harm" dictates that they be wary
of separating children from their families and engendering emotional trauma. On the other hand, the commitment to protect

This work originally appeared in the *American Journal of Orthopsychiatry* 56, April 1986.
Copyright © 1986 American Orthopsychiatric Association, Inc. Reproduced by permission.

children from harm precludes returning children thought to be in danger of further injury.

The dilemma is complicated by several other factors. In some cases the child may have sustained no traumatic injury, but his or her condition (e.g., severe neglect) may be a cause of concern. Where an injury has been sustained there is often a lack of clear information about how the injury occurred. Rational clinical judgment based on the child's condition and family circumstances may be difficult for clinicians because of an absence of systematically assembled data, anger and other emotions they may feel toward unprotecting parents, psychological denial, and culturally conditioned impressions of certain types of families.

Concern about the quality of alternative living arrangements for children removed from their homes further clouds decision making. Recent examinations of foster care have revealed the inadequacies, failures, and high costs of the system.[5,10,24] Although one might hope that foster care would provide a satisfactory *temporary* shelter while the family receives treatment, statistics suggest a different situation. The average length of time spent in foster care has been found to be about five years in some cities.[4] Moreover, more than half the children in foster care are moved to a new foster home at least once and are thus deprived of stable, continuous care giving.[15]

One way of allowing more children to return home is to provide troubled families with services that will strengthen the family unit. These may include traditional social services such as homemaker services, day care, or counseling. They may also include less official but equally important advocacy services such as working with landlords or welfare agencies on problems such as inadequate housing.[17] Providing support services may be a particularly appropriate alternative to removal in cases where the child's condition is not serious and the child does not appear at great risk. Indeed, several investigators have suggested that many children enter foster care due to problems such as family crisis or inadequate financial resources that could be better addressed by the provision of services.[7,8,14,21] Unfortunately such alternatives often are not considered or are unavailable.[14,18]

Despite the importance of the decision as to whether to remove a child, there has been little research on how such decisions are made. A growing body of research suggests that institutional biases affect decision making in child abuse cases. O'Toole and colleagues[20] found that physicians' judgments about whether abuse occurred in a set of emergency room vignettes were affected by the race and socioeconomic status of the family, as well as by level of injury. In a similar study, McPherson and Garcia[16] found that lack of familiarity with a family, but not low socioeconomic status, increased the likelihood of pediatricians diagnosing child abuse. Since minority and poor families are more likely to use emergency room facilities for their children's health care, and thus be unfamiliar to the physician, their findings are consistent with a greater proportion of poor families losing their children.

A study conducted by Hampton and Newberger[11] uncovered bias in the management of child abuse. In a national sample of suspected abuse and neglect cases, they found that hospitals tend to underreport white families to child protection agencies. Ninety-one percent of Hispanic and 74% of black families were reported to the child protection agency, while only 61% of white families were reported.

Studies of how child abuse is handled outside the medical system have also found that class, race, and other family characteristics affect decision making. Ross and Katz,[22] in a retrospective study of case records of a protective service agency, found that even after controlling for the nature of abuse, families receiving general welfare, families perceived by the agency as having a family member with a mental health problem, families with a child with behavioral problems, and families with a parent characterized as ineffectual were more likely to have a child removed. Runyan and colleagues[23] found that family characteristics such as substance abuse or an employed mother increased the likelihood of foster care placement, but that race and income were not significant predictors of placement. Studies of court decisions have revealed that factors such as substance abuse and the involvement of police may increase the likelihood that parents will lose their children in a court proceeding.[1,25] Thus a similar set of premises and biases that might lead professionals to identify and report certain families as abusers at an initial setting, such as a hospital, might subsequently influence decisions made about the fate of the family as it is channeled through the protective service and justice systems.

The current study examined the records of 185 suspected abused or neglected children seen at Children's Hospital, Boston, in an attempt to reveal how demographic characteristics, family history, family stress, the nature of the injury, and aspects of the medical encounter influence the outcome of the case.

Method

A coding instrument was developed and pretested to provide a standardized approach for reviewing the hospital records of children referred to the hospital's interdisciplinary child abuse consultation team, the Trauma X team. Data on the child, family, medical condition, and discharge disposition were obtained for each case. Each record was independently reviewed by two coders. Differences between coders were discussed in team meetings, and records were subsequently recoded to reflect the consensus of the study group.

Two hundred and eighty cases referred to the Trauma X team over a three-year period (1978–1981) were coded. This represented approximately 80% of the cases about which the Trauma X team was consulted and which fell within the official team review. The remaining cases were not coded because records were either incomplete or unavailable. Cases about which a Trauma X team member was consulted but which were not officially reviewed by the team were not coded because reliable data could not be obtained. (These tended to be emergency cases or unofficial consultations where all the decisions were made before the Trauma X team could meet.)

To be included in this analysis the child had to be living at home before hospitalization. Obviously, discharging a child to a foster home has a different meaning if the child was initially living in a foster home. In addition, only cases in which the child had sustained a physical injury (excluding animal bites) or in which there was a suspicion of neglect, failure to thrive, or poisoning were included in the analysis. Excluded from the analysis were cases in which the child had suffered a fatal injury or had been discharged to another hospital. (In this latter group of cases there was no analogous custody disposition.) These selection criteria resulted in a sample of 185 cases.

Family stress was measured using a checklist based in part on the Social Readjustment Rating Scale.[12] Stresses included on the checklist were death of a spouse, divorce, marital separation, jail term of parent or other household member, death of a close family member, pregnancy, death of a close friend, son or daughter leaving home, a handicapped child, unemployment, violence between spouses, and other significant stresses (up to two) present within a year of the current hospitalization. Items were added and grouped into two categories: families with no or only one stress (low stress) and families with more than one stress (high stress).

Two variables were used to characterize the nature of the injury. *Severity of condition* refers to the harm to the child's body or function. On a four-point scale the injuries were coded as: 1) life threatening, death imminent without medical intervention; 2) serious, death unlikely but further deterioration of function highly probable without medical intervention; 3) moderate, death or deterioration of function unlikely but the condition serious enough to interfere with usual function and treatment of some type necessary to hasten reversal of the injurious process; 4) minimal, possibility of slight loss of function, injury can resolve with or without medical intervention. *Physical injury* was coded as present if the child had an old or current physical injury (e.g., burn, laceration) or was suspected of being a victim of physical or sexual abuse. Cases of neglect, poisoning, and failure to thrive were coded as nonphysical injury. (Cases of physical injury with a nonphysical injury also present were coded as having a physical injury.)

Three case outcomes were distinguished: child returned home without services; child returned home with services; and child placed in foster home or institution. In cases in which the child was returned home ($N=37$), the decision was made that the family did not require further systematic intervention. These children were in most cases receiving medical follow-up through the hospital or other clinic, however. In cases in which the child was sent home with services, ($N=110$), services were provided on an ongoing basis; services included day care, homemaker, visiting nurse, therapy for child or family, or protective service involvement.

Out-of-home placements ($N=38$) included foster care with relatives or with nonrelatives, and residential placement. Some of the children in this group will subsequently be returned home, but even temporary removal may have a major impact on children and parents. Young children, in particular, may have difficulty understanding a "temporary" removal. For parents, a removal can be equally traumatic and undermine their sense of competence in caring for their children.

In many cases, actions by the protective service agency and the courts influence hospital management and discharge disposition. However, the opinions of professional reports such as medical personnel weigh heavily in the actions taken by protective service agencies[2] and the court. Moreover, to the extent that hospital clinicians make initial decisions regarding whether to file a report with the protective service agency or whether to seek court approval for custody, they choose the case of other professionals involved in the cases. It should also be noted that some of the placements of children outside the home may be "voluntary" by the parents.

Results

Sample Characteristics

Children ranged in age from one month to 16 years, with the sample skewed toward younger children (median = 16.3 months). Forty percent of the children were less than one year old and 70.8% were under three years of age. There were approximately equal numbers of girls (51.9%) and boys (48.1%).

The sample is composed predominately of lower-income families. Almost two-thirds of the families (65.4%) were eligible for Medicaid. Forty-two percent of the families were white, 36.4% black, 17.9% Hispanic, and 3.2% other ($N=184$). (The N is reported for all results where N is not equal to 185 due to missing data or a selected sample.) Over half of the families (52.8%) were female-headed households ($N=178$). The mean age of mothers was 26.3 (SD=7.2; $N=168$) and of fathers 29.7 (SD=8.3; $N=112$). Families had, on average, 2.3 children (SD=1.3), with 83.6% of families having no more than three children ($N=183$).

For a large number of families this was not their first contact with an agency due to concern about child maltreatment. Over one-fourth of the families (29.2%) were the subjects of reports to child protective services agencies either for the index child or for someone else in the family. Nineteen percent of children had a record of a previous accident ($N = 182$).

Commonly noted stresses included unemployment (47.0%), pregnancy (44.9%), and marital separation (23.8%). Seventy-one percent of families had more than one stress noted. This finding is in keeping with other research indicating a close association between family stress and child accidents and maltreatment.[3,6,13]

Eight percent of the conditions were rated as life-threatening, 35.9% as serious, 47.8% as moderate, and 8.2% as minimal ($N = 184$). These figures indicate that, while a substantial number of children sustain severe injury, the majority of cases are not severe. The wide range in severity of injury underscores the importance of having flexible responses to maltreatment cases.

In 73.5% of the cases, the child suffered a physical injury. The mother was suspected of maltreating or permitting maltreatment of the child in 44.3% of the cases in which a mother was present in the household ($N = 183$). In families in which a father was present, the father was suspected of being involved in the maltreatment in 40.7% of the cases ($N = 86$).

Forty-four percent of cases were seen through the medical emergency room and 39.2% through the surgical emergency room ($N = 176$). In almost all of the cases (97.3%), the child was admitted to the hospital; however, five cases (2.7%) were sent home after evaluation ($N = 184$).

Most of the children were cared for by a medical service (45.4%) or a surgical service (including neurosurgery, plastic surgery, and orthopedics) (50.2%), while the remaining patients were seen by the psychosomatic, outpatient, or other hospital clinic or service. The duration of stay for inpatients ranged from one to 169 days, with a median stay of 9.1 days ($N = 179$).

Analysis

We tested the influence of each independent variable on the outcome measure using χ^2 analyses. Results are presented in table D–1.

Table D–1
Independent Variables by Discharge Disposition

Variable[1]	Home	Home with Services	Out-of-Home
Medicaid Eligibility			
Yes (65.4%)	15.7%	59.5%	24.8%
No (34.6%)	28.1	59.4	12.5
$\chi^2 = 6.31$; $df = 2$; $p = .04$; ($N = 185$)			
Previous Filing			
Yes (29.2%)	9.3	50.0	40.7
No (70.8%)	24.4	63.4	12.2
$\chi^2 = 20.7$; $df = 2$; $p < .0001$; ($N = 185$)			
Race			
White (43.8%)	24.4	53.8	21.8
Black (37.6%)	19.4	61.2	19.4
Hispanic (18.5%)	9.1	69.7	21.2
$\chi^2 = 3.88$; $df = 4$; $p = .42$; ($N = 178$)			
Severity of Condition			
Life-threatening (8.2%)	26.7	53.3	20.0
Serious (35.9%)	16.7	66.7	16.7
Moderate (47.8%)	22.7	55.7	21.6
Minimal (8.2%)	13.3	53.3	33.3
$\chi^2 = 4.05$; $df = 6$; $p = .67$; ($N = 184$)			
Mother Involved in Maltreatment			
Yes (44.3%)	11.1	60.5	28.4
No (55.7%)	26.5	58.8	14.7
$\chi^2 = 9.51$; $df = 2$; $p = .009$; ($N = 183$)			
Father Involved in Maltreatment			
Yes (40.7%)	20.0	54.3	25.7
No (59.3%)	25.5	64.7	9.8
$\chi^2 = 3.87$; $df = 2$; $p = .14$; ($N = 86$)			
Physical Injury:			
Physical injury (73.5%)	23.5	59.6	16.9
Nonphysical inj. (26.5%)	10.2	59.2	30.6
$\chi^2 = 6.49$; $df = 2$; $p = .04$; ($N = 185$)			
Hospital Service			
Medical (47.5%)	11.9	61.9	26.2
Surgical (52.5%)	26.9	58.1	15.1
$\chi^2 = 7.81$; $df = 2$; $p = .02$; ($N = 177$)			
Emergency Room			
Medical ER (44.3%)	14.1	59.0	26.9
Surgical ER (39.2%)	24.6	65.2	10.1
No (16.5%)	27.6	44.8	27.6
$\chi^2 = 10.2$; $df = 4$; $p = .04$; ($N = 176$)			
Family Stress			
Low stress (29.2%)	33.3	44.4	22.2
High stress (70.8%)	14.5	65.6	19.8
$\chi^2 = 9.78$; $df = 2$; $p = .008$; ($N = 185$)			

Table D–1

Variable[1]	Home	Home with Services	Out-of-Home
Child's Age			
Under six (83.8%)	16.1%	62.6%	21.3%
Six or over (16.2%)	40.0	43.3	16.7
$\chi^2 = 8.99$; $df = 2$; $p = .01$; ($N = 185$)			
Previous Accident			
Yes (19.2%)	34.3	37.1	28.6
No (80.8%)	17.0	63.9	19.0
$\chi^2 = 8.83$; $df = 2$; $p = .01$; ($N = 182$)			

[1]Child's sex, mother's age, father's age, single mother, others present at home, and number of siblings at home were not significantly associated with discharge disposition.

Families who were Medicaid-eligible and those with a previous report of suspected child maltreatment were more likely to have their children removed. Minority families were not, however, more likely to lose their children.

Severity of condition was not significantly associated with outcome. Cases in which the mother was suspected of being involved in the maltreatment of the child were more likely to result in removal. (There was a similar trend when the father was suspected of being involved in maltreatment but the sample was small and the result was not statistically significant.)

The presence of a physical injury decreased the likelihood of a child being placed outside of the home. Over two-thirds of cases of physical injury (67.7%) were seen in the surgical service and 53.1% were seen in the surgical emergency room. It is not surprising, therefore, that cases involved with a surgical service, as well as those involved with the surgical emergency room, were also less likely to have a child removed.

Families in which the child was under the age of six and families that were experiencing more than one stress at the time of hospitalization were more likely to have their child sent home with services. Cases in which there was a history of a previous accident (which some clinicians might interpret as a possible abuse incident or sign that the family is under stress) were less likely to be sent home with services (more likely to be sent home without services or removed from their homes).

A severe limitation of bivariate analysis is that it does not tell us whether the predictor variables are independently associated with the dependent variable. To resolve this problem we employed log-linear analysis, which is a multivariate procedure for analyzing categorical data. We tested the influence of each key independent variable on the dependent variable, controlling for those independent variables that were significantly associated with the same discharge disposition in bivariate analyses as the key independent variable in question.

We found that the effect of class is not independent of a history of a previous report of child maltreatment, service type, or a mother's role in maltreatment. This finding does not mean that class is not important. Rather, it appears that more than a single effect is operating. There is a group of poor families that are more likely to have a history of a previous report ($\chi^2 = 5.96$; $df=1$; $p=.01$), be seen by the medical service ($\chi^2 = 7.16$; $df=1$; $p=.007$), and have the mother involved in the maltreatment ($\chi^2 = 10.6$; $df=1$; $p=.001$). Since these variables are strongly associated with poverty it is impossible to determine precisely why this group of cases is at risk for removal.

While we were unable to demonstrate an independent effect of class on discharge disposition, we found that there was a significant three-way interaction among class, presence of a physical injury, and discharge disposition (table D–2). Specifically, families that were Medicaid-eligible were more likely to have their child removed than were more affluent families in cases of physical injury and less likely to have their child removed in cases of nonphysical injury.

The history of a previous child abuse report was a significant determinant of placement outside the home, even after controlling for other independent variables.

In terms of those variables found to be associated with sending children home with special services, we found that the statistical effects of high stress and having preschool children are redundant. That is, either of the variables predicts to outcome, but neither variable has a unique statistical association with discharge

Table D–2
*Standardized Likelihood Deviates of Three-Way Interactions
with Discharge Disposition*[1]

Variable	Home	Home with Services	Out-of-Home
Nonphysical injury			
Medicaid eligible: Yes	.63	.23	– .67
Medicaid eligible: No	– 1.60	– .51	1.58
Physical Injury			
Medicaid eligible: Yes	– .33	– .16	.57
Medicaid eligible: No	.31	.19	– 1.02
$G^2 = 7.84^*$; $df = 2$; $p = .02$; $(N = 185)$			
Nonphysical Injury			
Low stress	1.08	.77	– 2.47
High stress	– .88	– .31	.85
Physical Injury			
Low stress	– .38	– .34	.97
High stress	.38	.20	– .84
$G^2 = 11.5^*$; $df = 2$; $p = .003$; $(N = 185)$			

[1]Residuals should be interpreted as deviations from the bivariate results (see table D–1). Positive numbers indicate a greater number of cases than expected in the cell, while negative numbers indicate fewer than expected cases in the cell.
*Results verified by random sampling.

disposition. This is consistent with the finding that families in which the child was of preschool age were under greater stress ($\chi^2 = 4.33$; $df = 1$; $p = .04$). There is a significant three-way interaction among family stress, physical injury, and discharge disposition (table D–2). While high stress increased the likelihood of going home with services in cases of physical injury, high stress increased the likelihood of removal in cases of nonphysical injury. Also, there is a marginally significant three-way interaction among family stress, previous report of child abuse, and discharge disposition ($G^2 = 5.59$; $df = 2$; $p = .06$), indicating that in low-stress families a previous report increases the likelihood of the child being returned home with services instead of home without services. High stress marginally increases the likelihood of a child returning home with services even after controlling for a history of a previous accident ($G^2 = 8.21$; $df = 4$; $p = .08$). Conversely, a history of a previous accident marginally decreases the likelihood of a child being returned home with services after controlling for family stress

($G^2 = 8.07$; $df=4$; $p=.09$). A three-way interaction among a previous accident, child's age, and discharge disposition ($G^2 = 10.84$; $df=2$; $p=.004$) indicates that preschool children with a previous accident are more likely to be removed, while older children with a previous accident are less likely to be removed.

Discussion

The data help us to understand those factors that do and do not influence discharge disposition of cases of abuse and neglect. We found that children with nonphysical injuries were more likely to be removed. One explanation for this result is that nonphysical injuries, which include failure to thrive and neglect, may be perceived by clinicans as evidence of chronic family problems rather than as a single mishap. Second, the decision to admit a child who does not have a physical injury (and therefore has more limited treatment possibilities) may itself indicate consideration of removal. A third possibility is that clinicans on the surgical services (which see the majority of children with physical injuries) are more likely to send children home after treatment than are clinicians on the medical services (which see the majority of nonphysical injuries).

While somewhat surprising, the fact that severity of condition was not associated with placement outside of the home is consistent with the findings of Hampton and Newberger.[11] It may be that, in considering whether to place children after hospitalization, other factors such as the perceived risk of reinjury to the child weigh more heavily in decision making. Alternatively, our scale of severity of injury may not be a sensitive measure. One important factor our scale does not take into account is the injurer's intention. A sharp object thrown at a young child may result in very different injuries depending on whether it just hits or just misses the child's eye. Yet the resulting injuries may be viewed similarly by clinicians who focus on the injurer's intention.

Social class was not found to have an independent effect on discharge disposition in the same as a whole. However, low-income families were more likely to lose their children in cases of physical injury. With physical injuries to young children it is difficult to establish whether the injury was inflicted or accidental. Indeed, several studies have suggested that accidents and abuse may have similar etiologies.[9,19] In clinical practice, however, physical injuries are open to two very different interpretations: abuse or accident. Our findings suggest that physical injuries may more frequently be diagnosed as "abuse" in poor families and more frequently characterized as "accidents" in more affluent families. The fact that more affluent families are more likely to lose their children in cases of nonphysical injury suggests that a negative evaluation is made of families who appear to neglect their children despite adequate financial resources.

Although, overall, clinicians took note of families that were under stress and provided them with services to maintain their integrity, multivariate analysis showed that this relationship was not true of cases of nonphysical injury in which high stress made removal more likely. One possible explanation for this finding is that families with chronic conditions, such as failure to thrive or neglect, and high stress are perceived as too overwhelmed to care for their child even with services. More intensive services, in addition to traditional protective service casework, such as freely available day care and homemakers, might allow more children to return home from the hospital.

A history of a previous child abuse report was an important determinant of placement outside the home. It may be that clinicians view these families as "repeat offenders," unable to protect their children. This finding should, however, remind us of the inherent dangers of labeling families as "child abusers" as occurs when there is a note in the child's medical record stating that the family was previously reported for abuse. Such a note may make further referrals to child protection agencies, as well as removals, more likely even when past reports may be unsubstantiated.

Two significant limitations of this study should be noted. First, it is an entirely hospital-based sample. Nonetheless, hospitalized children may be particularly at risk for removal because their injuries are generally more serious. Also, this sample reflects only those cases in which the Trauma X team was consulted, rather than all children entering the hospital who may have been abused or neglected. There was an initial "screening" of these cases before they reached the Trauma X team. This study cannot reveal the factors influencing the initial recognition of child abuse and neglect. While no bias against minority children emerged in this study, as it has in previous research,[11] white and minority children with similar conditions may not be referred to the Trauma X team in similar proportions.

Clinical Implications

Based on the findings of this study, as well as on the clinical experience of the child abuse team, we offer the following four recommendations.

1. *Formalize decision making.* Emotional reactions to cases are much more likely to affect case management if decisions are made by a single clinician on an ad hoc basis. This is true regardless of the talents or sensitivities of any individual clinician. A multidisciplinary group (including pediatrician, psychiatrist, psychologist, social worker, nurse, and laywer) offers an opportunity for involved clinicians to organize their observations about a particular case and receive feedback from a variety of perspectives.

2. *Include members of class and racial minorities in all decision-making groups.* One of the best ways to avoid bias in decision making is to ensure that there are members of the group who will represent the position of poor and minority families and who are especially sensitive to cultural differences in child rearing and family structure.

3. *Establish systematic linkages with social agencies.* The decisions made by hospital clinicians frequently require the support of other agencies, and particularly the state child protection agency. Close ties with social agencies will ensure the best service for the child.

4. *Act as advocates.* Clinicians must recognize and accept the important role they can play as advocates for their patients, both on a case-by-case and a community-wide basis. Clinicians must help families to obtain needed services so that their children can be safely returned home. Moreover, clinicians must also be advocates for governmental provision of services to troubled families so as to ensure that clinical judgments are not determined by the scarcity of services.

References

1. Aber, J. 1980. The involuntary child placement decision: Solomon's Dilemma revisited. In Child Abuse: An Agenda for Action, G. Gerbner, C. Ross, and E. Zigler, eds. Oxford University Press, New York.
2. Carr, A., and Gelles, R. 1978. Reporting Child Maltreatment in Florida: The Operation of Public Child Protective Service Systems. Report submitted to the National Center on Child Abuse and Neglect.
3. Daniel, J., Hampton, R., and Newberger, E. 1983. Child abuse and accidents in black families: a controlled comparative study. Amer. J. Orthopsychiat. 53:645–653.
4. Fanshel, D. 1981. Decision-making under uncertainty: foster care for abused or neglected children? Amer. J. Pub. Hlth. 71:685–686.
5. Fanshel, D., and Shinn, E. 1978. Children in Foster Care: A Longitudinal Investigation. Columbia University Press, New York.
6. Gil, D. 1970. Violence against Children. Harvard University Press, Cambridge, Mass.
7. Goldstein, J., Freud, A., and Solnit, A. 1973. Before the Best Interests of the Child. Free Press, New York.
8. Goldstein, J., Freud, A., and Solnit, A. 1979. Beyond the Best Interests of the Child. Free Press, New York.
9. Gregg, G., and Elmer, E. 1969. Infant injuries: accident or abuse? Pediatrics 44:434–439.
10. Gruber, A. 1978. Children in Foster Care. Human Sciences Press, New York.
11. Hampton, R., and Newberger, E. 1985. Child abuse incidence and reporting by hospitals: significance of severity, class and race. Amer. J. Pub. Hlth. 75:56–60.
12. Holmes, T., and Rahe, R. 1967. The social readjustment rating scale. J. Psychosomat. Res. 11:213–218.
13. Holter, J., and Friedman, S. 1968. Child abuse: early case finding in the emergency department. Pediatrics 42:128–138.
14. Keniston, K. 1978. All Our Children. Harcourt Brace Jovanovich, New York.
15. Knitzer, J., and Allen, M. 1973. Children without Homes: An Examination of Public Responsibility to Children in Out-of-Home Care. Children's Defense Fund, Washington, D.C.
16. McPherson, K., and Garcia, L. 1983. Effects of social class and familiarity on pediatricians' responses to child abuse. Child Welfare 62:387–393.
17. Morse, N., et al. 1977. Environmental correlates of pediatric social illness: preventive implications of an advocacy approach. Amer. J. Pub. Hlth. 67:612–615.
18. Newberger, E., and Daniel, J. 1976. Knowledge and epidemiology of child abuse: a critical review of concepts. Pediat. Ann. 5:15–26.
19. Newberger, E., et al. 1977. Pediatric social illness: toward an etiologic classification. Pediatrics 60:178–185.

20. O'Toole, R., Turbett, P., and Nalepka, C. 1983. Theories, professional knowledge, and diagnosis of child abuse. In The Dark Side of Families: Current Family Violence Research, D. Finkelhor et al., eds. Sage, Beverly Hills, Calif.
21. Ross, C. 1980. The lessons of the past: defining and controlling child abuse in the United States. In Child Abuse: An Agenda for Action, G. Gerbner, C. Ross, and E. Zigler, eds. Oxford University Press, New York.
22. Ross, C., and Katz, M. 1983. Decision Making in a Child Protection Agency. Unpublished manuscript, Yale University.
23. Runyan, D., et al. 1981. Determinants of foster care placement for the maltreated child. Amer. J. Pub. Hlth. 71:706–711.
24. Schor, E. 1982. The foster care system and health status of foster children. Pediatrics 69:521–528.
25. Weinberger, P., and Smith, P. 1970. The disposition of child neglect cases referred by caseworkers to a juvenile court. In Child Welfare Services, A. Kadushin, ed. Macmillan, New York.

For reprints: Eli H. Newberger, M.D., Children's Hospital, 300 Longwood Ave., Boston, MA 02115

References

American Humane Association. 1979. National analysis of official child neglect and abuse reporting. DHHS Publication No. (OHDS) 81-30232. Revised 1981.

Bittner, S., and Newberger, E.H. 1981. Pediatric understanding of child abuse and neglect. *Pediatrics in Review* 2(7):197.

Bourne, R., and Newberger, E.H. 1977. "Family autonomy" vs. "coercive intervention"?: Ambiguity and conflict in a proposed juvenile justice standard on child protection. *Boston University Law Review* 57(4):670–706.

———. 1980. Interdisciplinary group process in the hospital management of child abuse and neglect. *Child Abuse and Neglect* 4:137–144.

Bowles, R.T., Newberger, E.H., and White, K.M. 1985. Violence experienced by children: Issues of etiology for different manifestations. *Human Affairs* 8:1–17.

Buchanan, A., and Oliver, J.E. 1979. Abuse and neglect as a cause of mental retardation: A study of 140 children admitted to subnormality hospitals in Wiltshire. *Child Abuse and Neglect* 3:467.

Caffey, J. 1972. On the theory and practice of shaking infants: Its potential residual effects of permanent brain damage and mental retardation. *American Journal of Diseases of Childhood* 124:161.

Carr, A. 1977. Some preliminary findings on the association between child maltreatment and juvenile mistreatment in eight New York counties. *Report to the Administration for Children, Youth and Families: National Center on Child Abuse and Neglect.* Processed October 20, 1977.

Cohn, A.H. 1979. Effective treatment of child abuse and neglect. *Social Work* 24:513–519.

Cormier, B., Kennedy, M., and Sangowicz, J. 1962. Psychodynamics of father-daughter incest. *Canadian Psychiatric Association Journal* 7:203.

Costantino, C. 1981. Intervention with battered women: The lawyer–social worker team. *Social Work* 26:451–455.

DeMause, L., ed. 1974. *The History of Childhood.* New York: Psychohistory Press.

Finkelhor, D. 1979a. *Sexually Victimized Children.* New York: Free Press.

Finkelhor, D. 1979b. Social forces in the formulation of the problem of sexual abuse. Paper delivered at the Society for the Study of Social Problems Annual Meeting, Boston.

Fischhoff, J, Whitten, C.F., and Pettit, M.G. 1971. A psychiatric study of mothers of infants with growth failure secondary to maternal deprivation. *Journal of Pediatrics* 79:209–215.

Friedman, S.B., and Morse, C.W. 1976. Child abuse: A five-year follow-up of early case findings in the Emergency Department. *Pediatrics* 54:404.

Friedrich, W.N., and Boriskin, J.A. 1976. The role of the child in abuse: A review of literature. *American Journal of Psychiatry* 122(4):580–590.

Gagnon, J. 1965. Female child victims of sex offenses. *Social Problems* 13:176.

Garbarino, J. 1976. A preliminary study of some ecological correlates of child abuse: The impact of socio-economic stress on mothers. *Child Development* 47:178.

Gelles, R.J. 1974. *The Violent Home: A Study of Physical Aggression between Husband and Wives.* Beverly Hills: Sage.

———. 1976. Abused wives: Why do they stay? *Journal of Marriage and the Family* 38:659–668.

———. 1980. Violence in the family: A review of research in the seventies. *Journal of Marraige and the Family* 42:873–885.

———. 1981. Socioeconomic issues in child abuse. In Kerns, D.L., ed., *Child Abuse and Neglect.* Chicago: Saunders.

———. 1982. Applying research on family violence to clinical practice. *Journal of Marriage and the Family* 44:9–20.

Gil, D.G. 1970. *Violence against Children: Physical Child Abuse in the United States.* Cambridge: Harvard University Press.

———. 1975. Unraveling child abuse. *American Journal of Orthopsychiatry* 45:346.

Giovannoni, J.M., and Becerra, R.M. 1979. *Defining Child Abuse.* New York: Free Press.

Goode, W.J. 1971. Force and violence in the family. *Journal of Marriage and the Family* 33:624–636.

Green, A.H. 1978. Self-destructive behavior in battered children. *American Journal of Psychiatry* 135:5.

Greenberg, N.H. 1979. The epidemiology of childhood sexual abuse. *Pediatric Annals* 8:16.

Groth, N., and Birnbaum, J. 1978. Adult sexual orientation and attraction to underage persons. *Archives of Sexual Behavior* 7:175–181.

Hampton, R.L. 1983. Race, ethnicity, and child maltreatment: An analysis of cases recognized and reported by hospitals. Paper presented at the Groves Conference on Marriage and the Family, Freeport, Bahamas.

Harper, L.V. 1975. The scope of offspring effects: From caregiver to culture. *Psychological Bulletin* 82:784.

Hilberman, E., and Munson, K. 1977–78. Sixty battered women. *Victimology* 3(4):460–470.

Kempe, C.H, Silverman, E.N., Steele, B.F., Dragmueller, W., and Silver, H.K. 1962. The battered child syndrome. *Journal of the American Medical Association* 181:17.

Kinard, E.M. 1980. *Emotional development in physically abused children. American Journal of Orthopsychiatry* 51:686.

Klaus, M.H., and Kennel, J.H. 1976. *Mother-Infant Bonding.* St. Louis: Mosby.

Lustig, N., Dresser, J.W., Spellman, S.W., and Murray, T.B. 1966. Incest: A family group survival pattern. *Archives of General Psychiatry* 14:31.

Martin, H.P. 1980. The consequences of being abused and neglected: How the child fares. In Kempe, C.H., and Hefler, R.E., eds., *The Battered Child,* 3d ed. Chicago: University of Chicago Press.

Martin, H.P., and Beezley, P. 1977. Behavioral observations of abused children. *Developmental Medicine and Child Neurology* 19:373.

Milner, Joel S., and Ayoub, C. 1980. Evaluation of "at risk" parents using the child abuse potential inventory. *Journal of Clinical Psychology* 36:(4):945–948.

Nakashima, I.I., and Zakus, G.E. 1977. Incest: Review and clinical experience. *Pediatrics* 60:696.

National Center on Child Abuse and Neglect. 1981. Child sexual abuse: Incest, assault and sexual exploration. DHHS Publication No. (OHDS) 81-30166.

Newberger, E.H., and Bourne, R. 1978. The medicalization and legalization of child abuse. *American Journal of Orthopsychiatry* 48:593.

Newberger, E.H., Hagenbuck, J.J., Ebeling, N.B., Colligan, E.P., Sheehan, J.S., and McVeigh, S.H. 1973. Reducing the literal and human cost of child abuse: Impact of a new hospital management system. *Pediatrics* 51:840–848.

Newberger, E.H., Hampton, R.L., and White, K.M. 1986. Child abuse and pediatric social illness: An epidemiological analysis and ecological reformulation. *American Journal of Orthopsychiatry* 56:589–601.

Newberger, E.H., and McAnulty, E.H. 1976. Family intervention in the pediatric clinic: A necessary approach to the vulnerable child. *Clinical Pediatrics* 15(12):1155-1161.

Newberger, E.H., and Marx, T.J. 1982. Ecologic reformulation of pediatric social illness. Paper presented at the Annual Meeting of the Society for Pediatric Research, Washington, D.C., May 13, 1982.

Newberger, E.H., and Newberger, C.M. 1982. Prevention of child abuse: Theory, myth, practice. *Journal of Preventive Psychiatry* 1(4).

Newberger, E.H., Newberger, C.M., and Richmond, J.B. 1976. Child health in America: Toward a rational public policy. *Milbank Memorial Fund Quarterly* 54:249.

Newberger, E.H., Reed, R.B., Daniel, J.H., Hyde, J.N., Jr., and Kotelchuck, M. 1977. Pediatric social illness: Toward an etiologic classification. *Pediatrics* 60:178.

Parke, R.D., and Collmer, C.W. 1975. Child abuse: An interdisciplinary analysis. In Hetherington, M., ed., *Review of Child Development Research*, vol. 5. Chicago: University of Chicago Press.

Parker, B., and Schumacher, D.A. 1977. Battered wife syndrome and violence in the nuclear family of origin: A controlled pilot study. *American Journal of Public Health* 67(8):760–761.

Patterson, G.R., Reid, J.B., Jones, R.B., and Conger, R.E. 1975. *Families with Aggressive Children*, vol. 1. Eugene, Ore: Castalia Publishing.

Paulson, M.J., Abdelmonem, A.A., Chaleff, A., Thomasen, M.L., and Liu V.Y. 1975. An MMPI scale for identifying "at risk" abusive parents. *Journal of Clinical Child Psychology* 22–24.

Pfouts, J., and Renz, C. 1981. The future of wife abuse programs. *Social Work* 26:451–455.

Ponzetti, J., et al. 1982. Violence between couples: Profiling the male abuser. *The Personnel and Guidance Journal* 222–224.

Reidy, T.J. 1977. The aggressive characteristics of abused and neglected children. *Journal Clinical Psychology* 33:1140.

Rosenfeld, A. 1979. The clinical management of incest and sexual abuse of children. 1979. *Journal of the American Medical Association* 242: 1761.

Sarason, S.B., and Doris, J. 1968. *Psychological Problems in Mental Deficiency*, 4th ed. New York: Harper and Row.

Schneider-Rosen, K., Braunwald, K.G., Carlson, V., and Cicchetti, D. In press. Current perspectives in attachment theory: Illustration from the study of maltreated infants. In Bretherton, I., and Waters, E., eds., *Growing Points in Attachment Theory and Research*. Monographs of the Society for Research in Child Development.

Simrel, K., Berg, R., and Thomas, J. 1979. Crisis management of sexually abused children. *Pediatric Annals* 8:59.

Smith, S.M., Hanson, R., and Noble, S. 1975. Parents of battered children: A controlled study. In Franklin, A.M., ed., *Concerning Child Abuse*. New York: Churchill, Livingston.

Solomons, G. 1979. Child abuse and developmental disabilities. *Developmental Medicine and Child Neurology* 21:101.

Straus, M. 1977–78. Wife beating: How common and why? *Victimology* 2:443–458.

Straus, M.A., and Gelles, R.J. 1986. Societal change and change in family violence from 1975 to 1985 as revealed by two national surveys. *Journal of Marriage and the Family* 48:470–471.

Straus, M.A., Gelles, R.J., and Steinmetz, S. 1980. *Behind Closed Doors: Violence in the American Family*. Garden City, N.Y.: Doubleday.

Steele, B.F.C. 1978. The child abuser. In Kutash, I., Kutash, S., and Slesinger, L. (eds.) San Francisco: Jossey-Bass.

Summit, R., and Kryso, J.A. 1978. Sexual abuse of children: A clinical spectrum. *American Journal of Orthopsychiatry* 48:237.

Turbett, J.P., and O'Toole, R. 1980. Physicians' recognition of child abuse. Paper presented at the Annual Meeting of the American Sociological Association, New York.

Walker, L. 1977–78. Learned helplessness. *Victimology* 2:525–534.

Weinburg, K.S. 1955. *Incest Behavior*. New York: Citadel Press.

Weitzman, J., and Dreen, K. 1982. Wife beating: A view of the marital dyad. *Social Casework* 68:259–265.

Index

About the Authors

Kathy White is a full professor of psychology and chair of that department at Boston University. She is also director of the Family Research Training Program at BU, which is funded by the National Institute of Mental Health. Dr. White is coauthor of a textbook on family research methods that will be published in the fall of 1989.

Jane Snyder is on the faculty of the Massachusetts School of Professional Psychology and in private practice in Brookline, Massachusetts, where she works with children and families. She was the project evaluator of the Training Program on Family Violence at Children's Hospital in Boston.

Richard Bourne, J.D., Ph.D., is legal consultant to the Child Protection Program, Children's Hospital, Boston, and an associate professor of sociology at Northeastern University, Boston.

Eli Newberger is a pediatrician who became interested in child abuse and family violence in the course of his pediatric training at Children's Hospital in Boston. There, he organized the hospital's child abuse consultation program in 1970 and led efforts to develop a more substantial base for clinical practice. As director of the family development study he has made major contributions to the literature and to the development of sound programs, including the book *Critical Perspectives on Child Abuse*.

Please remember that this is a library book,
and that it belongs only temporarily to each
person who uses it. Be considerate. Do
not write in this, or any, library book.

DATE DUE

AP 04 '91			
MR 18 '91			
NO 20 '91			
ILL			
B-85			
4/15/92			
AP 27 '92			
NO 23 '92			
MY 16 '93			
ill 9-22 B733			
1/13/95			
APR 03 '97			
FE 27 '01			
MY 04 '07			